Containing the
Health Care
Cost Spiral

Containing the Health Care Cost Spiral

Mary Frances Callan, Ph.D.

David Clark Yeager

McGraw-Hill, Inc.

New York St. Louis San Francisco Auckland Bogotá
Caracas Hamburg Lisbon London Madrid Mexico
Milan Montreal New Delhi Paris
San Juan São Paulo Singapore
Sydney Tokyo Toronto

Library of Congress Cataloging-in-Publication Data

Callan, Mary Frances.
   Containing the health care cost spiral / Mary Frances Callan,
David Clark Yeager.
      p.   cm.
   Includes index.
   ISBN 0-07-009704-6 :
   1. Medical care—Cost control.   2. Insurance, Health—Cost
control.   3. Medical care—United States—Cost control.
4. Insurance, Health—United States—Cost control.   I. Yeager,
David Clark.   II. Title.
   RA410.5C34   1991
   338.4'33621—dc20   90-13235
                                                                CIP

1 2 3 4 5 6 7 8 9 0   DOC/DOC   9 5 4 3 2 1 0

ISBN 0-07-009704-6

*The sponsoring editor for this book was James Bessent, the editing supervisor
was Olive Collen, the designer was Naomi Auerbach, and the production
supervisor was Pamela A. Pelton. It was set in Baskerville by McGraw-Hill's
Professional Publishing composition unit.*

Printed and bound by R. R. Donnelley & Sons Publishing Company.

Contents

Preface

Nowadays, nearly every American business must deal with the complex and perplexing problem of health care benefits costs. The cost of many benefits programs has risen so dramatically in the recent past that many employers can no longer foot the bill. Consequently, employee medical benefits are being severely reduced or dropped altogether. The resulting increase in employee dissatisfaction can have severe and long-term financial effects for a company.

What, then, can employers do to contain the rising costs of medical benefits plans? One effective approach to containing medical benefit costs was designed in the late 1980s by the human resources department and employees of a public institution in the Rocky Mountain states. This approach, which requires the complete participation of all company employees from the CEO down, focuses on the concept of shared problem solving and shared responsibility. The institution found that only through a cooperative effort could significant cost-containment policies be initiated.

Containing the Health Care Cost Spiral is a book for everyone concerned about developing a sound, effective employee medical benefits program. The book is not a panacea for all that is wrong with the system. Significant changes in attitude, legislation, and social responsibility will be needed before the problems can be totally eliminated. Rather, this book proposes a framework that may be used to pull diverse employee and management groups together so that they can focus on a common problem and utilize both their own experiences and the experiences of other organizations to begin working toward a *reasonable* solution.

The book begins with an examination of the problem and a description of how the United States got to this point in its health care crisis. The focus of the book quickly narrows to a study of how the crisis is affecting U.S. businesses. The immediate steps taken by the Rocky Mountain institution mentioned above to control the run-away cost spiral are used as a basis for suggestions for other businesses interested in implementing similar formulas.

Acknowledging that taking immediate steps to control the problem may have short-term benefits, the book also recognizes that a thorough evaluation of a particular organization's health care benefit program is needed. A framework for initiating a detailed study and implementing the necessary changes is the major theme in *Containing the Health Care Cost Spiral*. Working with the appropriate consultants, insurance carriers, and health care providers, most organizations should be able to effectively implement the strategies described in the book and bring the health care cost spiral under control. Readers should be aware, however, in order to be truly effective, an approach must have been developed, promoted, and accepted within the organization in which it will be implemented.

As with most management strategies, the efforts that were made to bring health benefit costs under control cannot be abandoned once the new plan design is in place. Only effective and efficient monitoring and sustained effort by employers, employees, health care providers, insurance carriers, and consultants can contain costs and then hold them in check.

The authors wish to thank the following people for their continuing support and assistance: William Barnes, president, William T. Barnes Consulting, Bellevue, Washington; Dr. James Hager, superintendent, Beaverton School District, Beaverton, Oregon; Steve O'Dell, vice president and general manager, Lincoln National Health Plan of Colorado, Ltd., Denver, Colorado.

Mary Frances Callan
David Clark Yeager

Losing Control: Fighting the Steady Rise in Medical Benefits Costs

Japanese business and industry have received recognition in recent years for utilization of management principles that serve to improve quality and production. The Kaizen management theory asserts that quality is a direct result of continual involvement in the process of redesigning and refining production and operations.* This same principle can be applied to managing the present crisis in health care management which threatens to significantly disrupt employer-employee relations, company profits, and the structure of medical treatment in the United States. This crisis is everyone's problem and will require on-going development of cooperative solutions to bring it under control.

The Cost of a Healthy United States

What is the cost of keeping Americans healthy, and who should shoulder the expense? As recently as 25 years ago, routine medical care consisted of infrequent visits to (or from) the family doctor, hospitalization in severe cases of illness or trauma, and bed rest. Today, the nature of

*Masaaki Imia, *Kaizen: The Key to Japan's Competitive Success.* New York: Random House, 1986.

1

routine medical care has changed dramatically. Patients have come to expect highly technical services for the most ordinary ailments. Medical providers often refer patients to specialists, use a battery of diagnostic tests (many of which have only recently become available), and bring the patient back for several rechecks. It should come as no surprise that the cost of modern health care has risen dramatically.

The Reasons for Rising Medical Costs

The reasons for the astronomical increase in the cost of health can be found in several areas: technology is not inexpensive. The costs incurred in research and development of new medicines and diagnostic tools are passed on to the consumer. Physicians, faced with increased risk of malpractice suits, pass on the higher fees for malpractice insurance policies to their patients. At the same time, physicians strive to minimize the possibility of malpractice litigation by documenting diagnoses with as many tests and supporting opinions as possible.

Hospitals, which provide services prescribed by physicians for their patients, also provide services designed to reduce their exposure to malpractice litigation. Furthermore, many hospitals provide services to uninsureds and to indigents within the community, and pass such treatment costs on to the insured or paying consumer in an effort to balance their books. Patients make few decisions regarding their care once in the medical provider system. All these factors, taken together, indicate a problem that is growing out of control.

Rising Medical Care Costs: Who Pays the Bill?

Unfortunately, the cost of providing care to health-conscious Americans falls disproportionately upon U.S. employers and employees—not upon the medical community or insurance carriers. Insurance package programs such as managed health care, first-dollar coverage, and a myriad of "custom" benefit programs often do little to control costs. In fact, many of these programs have served to exacerbate the problem.

Strategies to Control Rising Medical Care Costs

This book provides a strategy for determining the specific needs of an organization and its employees, a logical approach for setting insurance procurement parameters, ways to effectively involve employees in decisions regarding health costs, and the tools necessary to negotiate effectively with insurance carriers and brokers. The book provides processes and strategies which have been developed and effectively used to control insurance costs. The strategies set forth here have been used effectively in organizations in which premium rates over a 3-year period would have reflected a 152 percent increase had the described management techniques not been employed. One public institution faced the possibility of having *no coverage* for its 2700 employees and dependents. By reducing some benefits and cost-shifting additional dollars onto the employee, that same increase was held to 34 percent, with a 0 percent premium increase for the year following the changes and an 11 percent increase for the succeeding year. It should also be noted that additional coverage was provided in areas considered to be most important by employee groups. Prescription and approval of the cost shifting and other additions by the employees themselves served to ease contract negotiations with employee groups, including unions that had previously opposed such changes in the members' benefits package.

There is no single approach to solving the problem of rising health care benefits costs. What is certain is that the problem is not going to go away on its own. Solutions can be achieved only with the full participation and consensus of senior staff, employees, and their representative associations in demanding responses from carriers and providers. Once solutions have been achieved, it is equally important to sustain the efforts and strategies that have been put into place.

The purpose of this book is to assist employers and employees to understand the problems associated with rising health care costs and with attempts to provide solutions. The book may anger some providers, be they doctors, hospitals, or carriers. Others may be pleased to discover that they will be working with informed consumers. Whatever the response, the approach described in the following pages will demonstrate that there is a way to control costs if everyone is willing to work together.

1
You Have a Problem

William Davis owns a small publishing company with 43 employees. In the last 5 years, he has seen the cost of health care benefits for his employees and their dependents rise over 150 percent. In order to contain the situation, he believes that he must choose one of three alternatives: (1) dramatically reduce the employees' benefits package, (2) shift more of the cost of coverage onto the employees, or (3) reduce the number of employees covered under the plan. Any of these solutions will have a negative effect on his ability to stay competitive in an aggressive marketplace.

Christine Dalton is human resources manager for a large metropolitan hospital. Since 1986, health benefits costs have risen a staggering 163 percent. While the hospital provides coverage for any employee working 20 or more hours per week, the cost of family coverage is the employee's responsibility. Many entry-level employees can no longer afford the premiums for family coverage; as a result, their dependents are uninsured. Sick leave, absenteeism, and low morale continue to increase proportionately with rising insurance premiums, thus adversely impacting negotiations with the hospital's employee unions.

Causes of the Deterioration of Medical Benefits

The situations described above are not unusual. Health care benefits costs are increasing throughout the country. Frequently, these costs cannot be absorbed by the employer and are passed on to employees through payroll deductions. Employees find themselves facing lower pay raises coupled with increased premium costs for plans that provide reduced benefits. Employee unrest spreads.

This spiral is affecting public and private institutions, Fortune 500 companies, and small proprietorships with equal devastation. Yet, awareness of the problem is only now beginning to spread. What was once regarded as an isolated series of events is now recognized as a per-vasive problem for which no simple solution is available. Every em-ployer in the country is currently dealing with the problem or will do so in the near future.

Early Detection: Deterioration Preceded by Four Warning Signs

Deterioration of medical benefits is usually a gradual process. However, if it is detected early enough, employers can implement several strate-gies for controlling costs. There are typically four signs of an impend-ing problem: an increase in premiums, a decline in covered services, a change in the manner in which provided services are recorded and paid, and a continual increase in the demand for medical services.

Premium Increases. The first sign of an impending problem with a medical benefits package comes when the current carrier proposes a premium which has increased over the annual inflationary factor for health care. This factor, called *trend*, continues to increase annually. For example, trend averaged 23.3 percent in 1989, and is projected to av-erage 20 percent in 1990.

Decline in Covered Services. A second sign of deterioration is noted when the health care services provided under the current benefits pack-age decline. Carriers begin to demand equal or increased premiums for reduced benefits. Employees discover that procedures that were once covered under old policies are no longer covered or are paid at a re-duced rate. Their dissatisfaction with the benefits program grows quickly.

Unbundling of Services. The third sign of deterioration often appears during a periodic utilization review of the benefits plan. A *utilization review* is an analysis of all costs charged to the plan and a breakdown by percentage for each type of service. *Unbundling of charges* occurs when services that providers once charged to a policy as a single item are broken into several separate charges. It is not unusual for unbundled services to total more than the insurance company's interpretation of "reasonable and customary" for the procedure. Although the premium continues to rise, fewer benefits are provided under the carrier's reimbursement interpretation, subtly shifting more of the financial responsibility for maintaining the plan to the employee.

Rising Demand for Medical Services.   Despite the increased personal cost, employees' use of medical services continues to increase, providing yet another indicator of impending trouble. Many employees have come to expect first-dollar coverage as well as small copayment provisions in the benefits package. Further, there now exists the expectation that a plan should cover more than medically necessary treatment, including, for example, cosmetic surgery, massage, and spa treatments. Such coverage, in turn, drives up usage. When use increases, plan costs quickly outpace employer premium contributions. The loss ratio is such that costs to the company begin rising dramatically. Table 1-1 shows how quickly, in the absence of cost-containment measures, costs can escalate; in this instance, 106.6 percent of the premium was spent on actual claims. When the ratio accelerates, medical benefit costs can become a serious drain on an operating budget, causing many companies to cut back on contracted services. Otherwise, the situation would quickly bankrupt the plan and result in significantly higher premiums.

Complications Precipitated by Legislative Action.   In addition, state and federal legislators often bow to powerful lobby groups and enact legislation that expands the coverage employers must provide. Mandated benefits may have a serious effect on employer-employee relations in the future if present costs are not brought under control.

How to Take a Stand

If your company is facing renegotiation of benefits within the next year or experiencing the effects of any of the conditions described above, several strategies presently available can reduce financial exposure and gain employee support. Rising medical benefits costs must be considered in the same light as any other internal cost issue. All members of the organization, from the maintenance crew to the chief executive officer (CEO) must be involved in interpreting the problem, identifying possible solutions, and acting in concert to reduce the drain on financial resources.

Table 1-1. Minimum Premium Group Paid Basis Report
1/1/87 to 1/1/88

Date paid	Premium	Monthly reimbursement deposit	Total funds	Paid claims	Ratio
1/1/87	$ 26,271.49	$ 207,984.36	$ 234,255.85	$ 227,114.04	97
2/1/87	25,130.37	206,002.62	231,132.99	265,079.57	94.7
3/1/87	26,085.35	206,263.66	232,349.01	203,221.65	87.5
4/1/87	26,401.17	208,812.41	235,213.58	224,803.89	95.6
5/1/87	26,359.02	208,485.58	234,844.60	253,246.65	107.8
6/1/87	26,263.06	207,740.27	234,003.33	269,717.15	115.3
7/1/87	25,601.48	202,498.71	228,100.19	204,588.40	89.7
8/1/87	25,732.28	202,399.53	228,131.81	290,703.82	127.4
9/1/87	26,544.07	191,923.61	218,467.68	317,792.24	145.5
10/1/87	26,074.17	224,299.76	250,373.93	222,892.47	89.0
11/1/87	27,044.95	214,173.03	241,217.98	190,232.20	78.9
12/1/87	26,584.71	209,542.12	236,126.83	319,493.71	135.3
Subtotal	$314,092.12	$2,490,125.66	$2,804,995.79	$2,988,995.79	106.6

Summary: Understanding the Problem

It is not uncommon for insurance premiums to rise at an annual rate of between 30 and 50 percent. In late 1989, Blue Cross and Blue Shield of Oregon requested from the state's Department of Insurance and Finance a 28.3 percent rate increase for holders of individual major medical insurance policies. According to several industry sources, medical care costs for individuals covered under a typical indemnity plan rose more than 20 percent in 1989, an increase of nearly 5 percent over 1988.

Who Designs the Policies You Purchase?

Insurance companies and independent brokers often design insurance benefits programs and sell them to a variety of companies without taking the time to first understand the individual needs and differences of the companies and their employees. Many of these "packaged" programs look effective on paper and may at first seem to be effective in use, because of the positive financial impact they appear to have on the benefits cost. But in reality, these programs merely shift costs to employees and reduce benefits. The net effect to the employer will be employee dissatisfaction, which quickly translates to increased internal problems. Rather than purchasing a solution, the employer may have unwittingly assumed a much larger problem. The responsibility for that problem remains with the organization and not the outside consultants, brokers, carriers, or providers.

The Origin of the Problem

Before you tackle the problem of increased benefits costs, it is important to understand its origins. Medical costs, which at one time represented a small portion of the gross national product (GNP), now represent more than 11 percent. Medically related services collect in excess of $500 billion annually. Supply companies will continue to grow into the next century. Today, a variety of consumer-oriented technologies are available to both the general practitioner and the specialist. The result has revolutionized health care, but the cost-benefit issues surrounding these new technologies have not yet been adequately addressed.

The Role of the Federal Government. The role of the federal government in medicine has increased beyond the stage of research funding.

Today, several government agencies are directly involved in designing and pricing services (e.g., Medicare and Medicaid), controlling the nature and distribution of medical supplies (Food and Drug Administration and Drug Enforcement Administration), as well as proposed taxation of benefits to highly compensated employees [Section 89 of the Internal Revenue Code (IRC)]. Although Section 89 was repealed, many insurance analysts believe that the issue of taxation of benefits will remain under consideration. In addition, many congressional representatives are concerned with delivery of medical care services to uncovered employees and indigents within their constituency. Myriad legislative restraints that could dramatically affect the delivery of health care services and their costs have been proposed and are now pending.

Who Is Responsible?   As all these factors come into play, the cost of insuring employees becomes greater and the hope of budgeting for future increases becomes impossible. Containing the cost of doing business is essential for any organization, public or private. Successful containment of rising medical costs will never be accomplished by insurance companies, outside brokers, or government officials alone.

In addition, the management team within each organization is responsible for designing and maintaining a process of continual evaluation and improvement of the health benefits program and for demanding appropriate responses from the health care industry and its providers. This is a responsibility that employers cannot shirk unless they are willing to throw out all control over their medical benefits plans and rely upon the federal government to debate, construct, enact, and mandate an insurance program to be paid for through employer contributions.

The following section outlines the issues that must be examined. Subsequent chapters will assist in providing the answers.

Focus Guide

In examining the current state of your benefits program, the answers to the questions below are essential for making practical decisions.

Cost Analysis

- Where are the dollars you place into the benefits program going?
- Where have the increases occurred?

- What are the areas of heaviest use?
- What changes can be made that will most dramatically cut costs while still providing effective coverage?

Employee Participation

- How can you effectively involve employees in helping to control the cost of the benefits program?
- How can managers assist in helping employees understand the problem?
- What types of information need to be provided to employees?
- How can you gain and maintain the trust of employees?
- What parameters need to be put into place that will be accepted by both management and employees so that solutions to the problem can be effectively examined?
- How can you best determine employees' needs in relation to their coverage?

Outside Assistance

- Is it necessary to bring in an outside consultant?
- What type of consultant best fits your company's need?
- How do consultants work with management and employee teams?
- What is the consultant's relationship with the insurance companies?
- What type of training does your team need to remain independent of the consultant?
- How do you make certain that the company's interest and the employees' needs will be met through the consultant's proposals?

Developing Solutions

- How do you determine employee and management needs?
- How do you analyze these needs?
- How do you assess the cost and potential impact of the solutions?
- Where and what are the trade-offs of each proposal?
- What impact will your proposed solutions have on in-force insurance packages?

- What is the impact on your tax exposure and that of your employees?
- How much change are your employees willing to assume?

Presenting Solutions

- How do you explain the proposed solutions to your staff?
- How do you effect major or minor modifications based on employee concerns?
- How do you involve the health care community, the consultants, and the insurance companies in effecting your plan?

Implementing the Solutions

- What changes need to be made in your present plan?
- Is the entire benefits package in need of restructuring?
- What questions and concerns will your employees raise?
- Do you have answers? How can you anticipate employee concerns?

Monitoring and Adjusting

- What procedures do you have in place to fine-tune the program?
- What procedures need to be developed?
- How do you plan to monitor the effectiveness of changes?
- What ongoing employee involvement do you have in place?
- How do you plan to meet counterproposals from the insurance company and health care providers within the community?

The process implied by the preceding questions is familiar to employers and mangers concerned about the continuing improvement of their company and their products. However, it is not common for this process to be applied to the problem of employee medical benefits. And yet, it should be applied to this problem. Increasingly, employers and managers are turning to insurance industry representatives to solve what is both an internal and an external problem. The result is a partial, if not total, abdication of control over benefits programs. The consultants retained by the company to solve the benefits problem often stand to profit the most through commissions, fees for service, and accounting services. The end result may not be cost containment.

Consumer Concerns

Individual subscribers should also be closely examining the benefits provided by their group policy, and asking pertinent questions.

- Has the amount of money that I pay toward my medical insurance benefits increased in the last year?

- Are the benefits presently provided by the policy the same as in previous years, or have these benefits increased or decreased over time?

- Is filing a claim with the carrier an easy task, or has the amount of red tape recently increased?

- Has my dependence upon my group health insurance decreased, increased, or remained fairly constant over the past year?

2

Getting a Handle on the Problem

In Search of Health

Rising health care costs have become a national issue. Americans' passion for fitness and youth has created a strong demand for medical treatment that can provide, or give the illusion of providing, every medical consumer with a clean bill of health. Americans spend a far greater amount on medical treatment than do citizens of other nations. In fact, according to recent estimates, Americans spend twice as much for medical treatment as the Japanese, and three times as much as the British. As Americans are not demonstrably healthier than the Japanese or British, they may not be getting an adequate return on their investment.

Medical Benefits Costs Have a Direct Effect on Profits

Every employer offering coverage to employees is affected by the growing demand for medical services and their dramatically increasing costs. If a business is to survive, the employer must develop an understanding of the problem and a strategy for dealing with it. These rising costs and the factors that contribute to them have become and will continue to be a drain on profits. Within the past few years, American corporations have been forced to shoulder an ever-increasing share of doctors' bills. Medical benefits costs alone are close to 14 percent of total payroll.

Most employers not directly involved in the medical care industry are not in a position to know all the ramifications of the problem, but they must develop a working knowledge of medical care costs so that informed decisions about employee coverage can be made. The effect of these decisions on short- and long-term profits must be realized. While such a commitment will require many hours of management and staff attention, the alternative will soon become unacceptable.

Seeking Outside Advice

There are those who would contend that it is not in the best interest of a company to invest large amounts of staff time and money researching medical benefits when outside "experts" are available. These experts range from brokers and consultants to insurance carriers and health care providers, all of whom are willing to design and implement medical insurance programs for employers and their employees. While outside consultants are able to provide a perspective, it is essential that employers perceive the problem of rising employee benefits costs in the same light as they would any other internal problem affecting profit or product. It is unlikely that any employer would be willing to abdicate his or her decision-making power about any other internal problem to a consultant. And yet, that is precisely what is happening when employers face problems with their employee medical benefits program.

Who Works for Whom?

Many employers are accepting the advice and counsel of experts from the medical care industry in selecting and implementing their medical care program. Yet, these brokers or consultants may not always be working exclusively for the client. Like any business person, the consultant must develop strong working relationships within the industry. These relationships can include, but are not limited to, physicians organizations, insurance brokers and companies, data processing and case management services, as well as other consultants. While these relationships are not in themselves detrimental, it is necessary to clarify any ambiguity. Are you really the client, or is the consultant representing one or several insurance carriers?

Many insurance brokers are willing to help employers select a medical insurance carrier on a no-fee basis. Initially, this arrangement appears to be cost-effective to the employer since little money is being spent for the consultation. The employer has found someone with a working knowledge of insurance programs and costs. Every question seems to have an answer, and the most difficult questions are often addressed with a reassuring, "Why don't you leave that to me?" The problem of employee medical benefits seems to be solved.

Look Closely at "Packaged" Programs

Unfortunately, a benefits package developed by a broker does not always serve the best interests of the employer or the staff. It is important to remember that someone is paying the expenses incurred by the broker. Many brokers are receiving between 2 and 5 percent of the cost of the plan they provide to the employer. This cost is included in the retention portion of the insurance premiums paid by the employer and employees as administrative charges.

This is not to say that employers should not make use of outside brokers and consultants when it is appropriate to do so. But the information these people supply should be evaluated and used in the context of the specific needs of the organization—and one of those needs is to control spiraling costs of employee benefits. Ultimately, it will be the employer and not the consultant who will have to maintain control over how insurance benefit dollars are to be spent.

How the Premium Dollar Is Spent

An employer can expect 75 to 80 cents of every premium dollar to be spent on the medical expenses covered under the plan. About 6 to 10 cents should go toward administration of the plan (processing claims, writing checks, preparing employee booklets and ID cards, and overhead). These administrative costs are referred to as *retention*. The remaining approximately 10 to 19 cents is used to build up a reserve fund to cover claims that are *incurred but not reported* (IBNR) when the plan year ends and to provide coverage for individuals who will be covered under the *extension of benefits* (EOB) provisions when the plan is terminated. Typically, EOB provisions provide continued coverage for individuals who are disabled at the time the plan terminates. The length of time during which these EOB provisions apply is determined by contract language, and this coverage applies only to disabled insureds who have no other coverage. The definition of disability can vary from one plan to another, but typically applies to insureds who are unable to continue or return to work.

The First Year of Coverage

Whenever a new insurance plan is enacted, the base of the reserve fund is built during the first year, thereby reducing the actual amount of money that can be spent on covered medical expenses. Since the total amount of the reserve fund must only equal 15 to 25 percent of the total premium dollar, less money has to be placed in reserves in succeeding years. The size of the reserve depends upon projected IBNR and EOB provisions. Since the reserve continues to grow each year a plan is in effect, the size of the reserve can eventually exceed what is necessary to cover IBNR and EOB provisions. The reserve can then be used to stabilize rising premiums and to cover unexpected costs.

Plan Ratings

Another source of confusion for many employers that are attempting to redesign their benefits plans is how those plans are rated by insurance carriers. There are two common ratings: experience-rated and community-rated.

1. *Experience-rated.*   With a premium that is experience-rated, the cost of the premium is determined by the costs of your group. Medical care, as paid out by the carrier, is totaled and added to the retention, reserve, and trend costs. The gross amount is then divided by the total number of insureds to arrive at a premium. In experience-rated plans, it is possible to monitor the costs of the plan for a specific group.

2. *Community-rated.*   If the plan is community-rated, then the costs of all individuals enrolled in that plan—including the employees not in your organization—are totaled to determine the premium cost.

A major disadvantage of community rating is found in an employer's inability to determine what is driving up insurance costs in general and his or her annual premium in particular. With most community-rated plans, since everyone who is covered under the plan is used to quantify and qualify costs, it is difficult to obtain specific information on the employees of a single organization. Because the information is unavailable, employers and employees in a community-rated plan cannot monitor their actual costs by reviewing their claims experience.

Medical Trend

While the costs described above serve as the basis for premium pricing, the factor of trend causes the rate structure to increase. Trend is made up of several things: the rise in the medical consumer price index, cost shifting and averaging of costs, new advances in medical technology, and increased utilization of medical care services. All these conditions have a direct impact on the charges incurred by the patient during the most routine physician's visit.

Trend as an Accelerator of Premium Costs

In the late 1970s and early 1980s, trend was rather slight and added between 4 and 8 cents to each annual premium increase. Today, trend is expected to run at 20 percent for 1990 and may go higher because of the recent repeal of catastrophic coverage for Medicare subscribers.

Therefore, a medical benefits plan that spends only 75 to 80 percent of the premium on actual medical expenses can show dramatic annual increases. Often, these annual increases in premium run much higher than the actual trend figure. During the last few years, it has not been unusual to see premium increases running anywhere from 30 to 50 percent. Insurance carriers present this trend to their customers in the most positive light, stressing among other things the benefits of improved medical technology.

The Uninsured

What seems to be the underlying cause for this increase in medical care costs? One disturbing factor is the tremendous growth in the number of individuals and families who carry no health insurance at all. Sixty percent of the uninsured in this country are employed and as a result of their employment are above the poverty line. It has been found that many uninsured individuals are reluctant to seek medical treatment until their illness becomes so severe that it cannot be ignored. As a result, the medical care they require is more complex—and more expensive.

Many expectant mothers who are uninsured do not receive any prenatal care prior to arriving at a hospital for delivery. The lack of a solid prenatal program increases the likelihood of complications at birth or medical problems for the infant. The need for greater recuperation time and physician care increases the costs. While most communities have hospitals and doctors who provide care to the indigent, this care is not free. The costs are passed on to the paying consumer in the form of increased medical charges. Until the issue of medical insurance coverage for the uninsured is resolved, the costs will be passed on to those who are covered or have the ability to pay. Indications are that by the turn of the century nearly 25 percent of the nation's current 6800 hospitals may have to close their doors. Hardest hit will be publicly subsidized and nonprofit hospitals, as they treat the largest percentage of uninsureds.

The Graying of the United States

America's aging population also is having a profound effect on the both the structure and delivery of medical services. Americans are living longer and maintaining a higher quality of life. The costs associated with keeping an aging population healthy are spread throughout society. This is also serving to raise ethical questions. For Americans who work later in life, as well as for retirees covered under former employers' insurance, the cost of medical security is often reflected in the employers' benefits costs.

Advanced Medical Technology

Advanced medical technology has added a broad new vocabulary to the lexicon of science. It has also served to dramatically drive up the cost of medical service. Transplants, laser surgery, lithotripters, and magnetic resonance imaging (MRI) are medical advances that promise longer, healthier lives. And they must be paid for. The costs of technological acquisition are passed on directly to the consumer. In communities where the health care providers have collectively purchased expensive state-of-the-art MRI equipment, there is a corresponding perceived need for its use, even though computerized axial tomography (CAT) scans and X rays might serve the same purpose at a fraction of the cost of the average MRI.

The Ethics of Technology.   While medical technology has been able to protect and prolong life, it has also prompted raging ethical debates. For example, current neonatal technology makes it possible to increase the survival rate of 1-pound premature infants. A few years ago such children died within a few hours of birth. Some preemies have been able to survive for as long as a year through the use of advanced technology, typically at a cost of more than $1 million each. It should not escape attention that most medical insurance plans have a $1 million maximum lifetime benefit. When that maximum is reached, insurance benefits stop, and providers often inform the parents that without the use of continued extraordinary methods, there is no hope for the child. Few parents have the financial resources to continue the life-support methods. A painful decision then follows. While continued use of these neonatal techniques may one day ensure the continued existence of a 1-pound infant, the cost for this potential advance is now being borne by those who are covered by medical insurance or who are able to pay.

Increased Medical Competition.   Another factor contributing to higher medical costs is the excess supply of medical care providers. Oversupply intensifies competition and stimulates the availability and use of medical services. The number of physicians graduating from medical school will continue to increase through the beginning of the next century. Advertisements for medical services continue to proliferate on prime-time television, notably in the area of adolescent psychiatric services. Once again, ethical questions about the effectiveness of these procedures can be raised, but this approach to increasing patient loads is undeniably profitable for the providers.

Rising Fee Structures. Despite increased competition, the fees charged by physicians for their services continue to rise. Ironically, development of negotiated price arrangements that offer fixed or discounted prices to patients who enroll in health management organizations (HMOs) and preferred provider organizations (PPOs) appears to have created additional price pressure in the fee-for-service market. Even with negotiated price arrangements, it is not uncommon for a family practitioner to earn $150,000 a year. In the late 1980s the increase in physicians' net incomes outpaced their increased expenses. Naturally, passing the increased expenses on to the consumer is justifiable. What is perplexing, however, is an additional double-digit increase in fees for the same period which cannot be attributed to increased expenses.

Elective Surgeries. Further, many of the operations being prescribed by physicians are of questionable necessity. Each year, thousands of women are subjected to unnecessary hysterectomies. Coronary bypass surgeries are performed on patients who do not need them. Until some way is found to halt unnecessary and expensive surgical procedures, the cost of medicine in this country will continue to rise.

The failure to recognize that limited resources are available to pay for medical care before other priorities are effected has taken its toll. These factors indicate that pressure on medical care costs will continue long into the future. Attempts to significantly control rising medical care costs appear to have failed. Certainly, a solution can be found, but it will require the cooperation of everyone involved in the problem: employers, employees, providers, insurance carriers, and consultants. Everyone must be willing to make some compromise—give up some level of profit or comfort in an effort to control costs.

The Effect of State and Federal Regulations

Federal regulations have also caused employers' medical care costs to soar. These regulations include the Consolidated Omnibus Budget Reform Act (COBRA), which mandates that employers must allow former employees and their dependents to continue purchasing group insurance for up to 36 months after leaving the job. This ceiling may soon be raised to 5 years. Employed individuals must pay into the Medicare fund through an employee payroll tax. In addition, they are charged a second time for this federally mandated program when the health care provider passes on to the insured those costs not covered by Medicare. Congress has proposed requiring employers to report the cost of covering benefits for future and current retirees on the annual balance sheet.

Mandated Benefits Programs

In recent years both federal and state governments have mandated a variety of health care coverage programs. This mandated health coverage has, for example, made pregnancy an illness, thereby driving up the cost of prenatal and postnatal care. When maternity and pregnancy coverage were not treated as an illness, but rather as a condition for which a lump sum would be paid unless there were aggravating conditions, costs were stabilized. Once pregnancy came to be treated as an illness, costs escalated. It became possible to treat each service separately and unbundle the fees for services and procedures. Adding to this is the high cost of malpractice insurance for obstetric and gynecological care. Medical coverage for nervous disorders has also been mandated in many states. This has served to increase the number of practitioners as well as the costs of services.

Ironically, as mandated services proliferate, the interpretation of what is covered and what is not becomes more strict. This has served to cause a lack of coverage for some medical techniques that might be available to deal with the same condition. Conversely, some of the services mandated by state and federal regulations appear not to be medically necessary. One classic example occurs in Minnesota, where health plans are required to offer hair replacements for covered individuals who have alopecia areata, a disease that causes hair loss. The prevailing philosophy seems to be that if some benefit may be derived from a procedure, it should be prescribed regardless of the cost. This philosophy needs to be examined in light of the increasingly limited financial resources available to cover such procedures.

Since the late 1960s hundreds of medical benefits have been mandated. While many of these benefits, such as newborn care and benefits extended to handicapped and adopted children, appear to be appropriate, they nonetheless have served to increase the costs of coverage. Escalating costs attributed to mandated coverage have driven many large employers away from benefit programs. Many of them have turned to self-insurance, which allows them to escape the mandated benefits under the Employee Retirement Insurance Security Act (ERISA). Obviously, this is not an option for small employers that cannot afford to plan for or absorb unanticipated costs. Therefore, small employers either must continue to provide mandated benefits in their packages or must reduce or drop coverage entirely.

Many mandated benefits were enacted at the urging of health care providers and their various associations. It now appears that, while some short-term benefit may have been derived from mandates, the long-term effect may be detrimental. If the current course is followed, the ultimate mandated program—a national health care program for all citizens—may become a reality. If this occurs, medical care providers may experience a significant loss of latitude in their approach to medicine.

Who Are the Players?

Responsibility for contributing to rising medical benefits costs cannot be placed on any single individual or group. The people responsible are in the ranks of providers, brokers and consultants, insurance carriers, employers, and employees throughout the nation. Many insureds have grown to expect first-dollar coverage and physicians' services for every cold and runny nose they contract. Most are unwilling to cut back on those services. At the same time, the medical providers seem unwilling to consider the issue of "overdoctoring" for fear of resulting malpractice charges. The legal profession continues to press malpractice claims, and most insurance carriers continue to pass on the costs to the consumer, acting merely as conduits for premium dollars rather than becoming actively involved in the solution through cost management, utilization review, or managed care. Collectively, insurance carriers, medical providers, and lawyers continue to lay the blame at the feet of the consumer who is demanding care.

Cost-Containment Strategies
Initiated by Carriers and Providers

If the current trend continues, medical care costs in the United States may constitute more than 15 percent of the gross national product

(GNP) by the year 2000. As the premiums have continued to spiral upward, some health care providers and insurance carriers have initiated cost-containment practices. The most common cost-containment practices endorsed by these groups provide for negotiated price arrangements. Most notable among these strategies is the growth of HMOs, exclusive provider organizations (EPOs), and PPOs.

Provider Organizations.   The manner in which these organizations work with their patients serves to distinguish one organization from the other. An individual enrolled in an HMO must first see a primary care physician. This physician acts as a gatekeeper, referring the patient to a specialist only if necessary. EPOs also use the physician gatekeeper, although the physician referral network is generally much smaller than that of an HMO. PPOs are often less structured than the other two groups. Patients using a PPO may enter the system at any point without seeing a gatekeeper. All the groups place insureds in a small physician network whose providers have agreed to take lower fees in exchange for a higher patient load.

Negotiated Price Arrangements.   Some of these negotiated price arrangements have resulted in capitated fees, most commonly found in HMOs. Under a capitated fee structure, physicians accept a flat fee for each person enrolled in their plan. If the value of the services used by the patient is less than the annual fee and overhead, this difference is provided to the physician in the form of a bonus. The capitated fee structure raises obvious ethical questions about the quality of patient care. For whom are individual physicians working? Themselves, or the provider organization to which they belong? What advantages flow to the patient who sees a physician affiliated with one of these organizations? Does such a system assure a better quality of care?

Continued Increase in Cost-Containment Practices

The number of industry-designed cost-containment procedures increases annually. In recent years, providers and insurance carriers have begun to require patients to use generic drugs, to accept home health care as an alternative to long-term hospitalization, and to undergo precertification and preadmission procedures prior to hospitalization. More aggressive cost-containment procedures limit benefits for weekend admissions and for overnight admissions prior to surgery in nonemergency cases, require detailed audits of hospital and doctor bills, and insist upon individual case management by either the carrier or a third-party organization.

Elimination of First-Dollar Coverage. Most notable among cost-containment strategies designed by insurance carriers is the proposal to eliminate first-dollar coverage and thus shift a greater portion of the cost onto the insured. While some would argue that increasing the dollar amount for which the patient is responsible will drive the sick away from their doctors, there is little evidence to support that position. A recent Rand Corporation study concluded that there is no appreciable difference in the health of patients with higher deductibles. What the higher deductible does is to make the patient a more health-conscious consumer.

Despite containment strategies, the cost of health care coverage continues to increase. The proliferation of restrictions initiated by insurance companies has not been met with a corresponding decline in the demand for services. Americans seem willing to work through a maze of restrictions and requirements in search of medical service.

Code Creep

Further complicating the problem are two billing techniques that physicians may use to circumvent cost-management procedures. The more commonly used billing practice, "code creep," occurs after a patient has come in for an office visit. At the end of the appointment, the physician places a code on the patient's bill, indicating such things as whether the examination was limited or comprehensive and whether the patient was new or established. The coded bill is then submitted to the insurance carrier either by the patient or directly by the doctor.

The codes used for these office visits are found in *Common Procedures Terminology* (4th edition)[*] and are referred to as CPT4s. A 90050, for example, is common for a routine office visit by a patient who has seen the doctor previously, whereas a 90070 is a code for an extended visit. Since the inception of PPOs and EPOs, insurance carriers have noticed code creep: office visits in the 90050 category have dropped while 90070 office visits have increased. Obviously the cost of an extended office visit is greater than that of a limited visit, therefore bringing in more cash for the physician. Additionally, PPOs and EPOs that require patients to make a small copayment, such as $5 or $15, for

[*]American Medical Association, Chicago, 1989.

each office visit have encouraged an increase in usage by patients. This situation, combined with code creep, defeats the purpose of cost management.

Unbundling

The second billing practice that leads to escalating medical costs was actually introduced by Medicare, which requires physicians to price separately certain items such as injections. While an injection might previously have been billed as a single procedure, the cost of that injection under unbundling would include a tray fee, a needle fee, and a serum fee. Medicare requested this in order to prevent overcharging for the serum. Unfortunately, unbundling has led to a proliferation of additional charges that insurance carriers had not seen previously. One carrier noted that, for example, some surgeons are charging separately for an incision, for removal of an organ, and for examination of the region around the removed organ to ensure that surrounding tissues are all right. Unbundling increases the number of areas in which charges can be made. Code creep, unbundling, and increased office visits can render many cost-management procedures useless unless these cost-management procedures are continually monitored and evaluated to determine whether they remain financially and socially responsible.

The Gauge Corporation: The Unwanted Effects of Adding a PPO

In 1986 The Gauge Corporation offered its employees a new insurance plan that included a PPO. The PPO provided for a $5 patient copayment for office visits to physicians who participated in the insurance carrier's plan. Within 3 years, the number of physician visits by employees doubled, code creep and unbundling appeared, and the plan was nearly bankrupt. While the carrier's cost-management program did reduce the number of inpatient surgeries, it could not contain the number of surgeries being performed in outpatient settings.

Although the carrier's policies were designed to decrease the cost of medical care, they actually drove costs up, due in part to the increase in outpatient surgeries and in part to a corresponding increase in bed charges as the number of filled beds declined because of the outpatient surgeries. In response to the failure of many of its cost-management practices, Gauge's carrier proposed reducing the benefits that would be paid, shifting more of the cost of the program onto employees, and increasing premiums.

Not surprisingly, employees at Gauge were outraged. Rather than sharing some of the blame for the situation, they felt abandoned and disenfranchised by both their employer and the insurance carrier. The Gauge Corporation and its employees had lost more through the initiation of the PPO than they gained.

The example above demonstrates some of the problems associated with initiating a new insurance package without careful planning and implementation. As this situation is multiplied hundreds of times across the nation, consumer groups, political assemblies, and employee bargaining units have begun to demand solutions. In fall 1989 several national employers were hit with strikes. One of the major unresolved issues was employee health care benefits. A possible solution to this discontent would be establishment of a national health care policy which would place all citizens under a single plan, or within large HMOs.

Summary: Understanding the Problem

Although, as stated above, a national health care plan would be one solution to current health care problems, less dramatic alternatives are currently available to employers. These alternatives can enable employees to retain a level of choice in medical decisions. If controlling the rising cost of medical care coverage is a priority, then it is necessary to design a program that fits the unique needs of employees and their dependents and which also includes provisions for managed care. Program design is not a simple, one-step process. It requires employer and employee education, participation, and shared decision making. A factor that must be recognized is that, whatever is done, rates will likely continue to rise. However, the *rate* of premium increase can be controlled. Employee benefits may be reduced or premiums may be increased, but through thoughtful benefit program design, it is possible to avoid having both happening simultaneously.

When designing a new health care plan, employers are often uncertain how best to approach the issue. The best place to begin is by examining where current dollars are being spent for medical care coverage. Everything about the current plan must be examined. The section below will assist you in examining the essential issues covered in this chapter.

Focus Guide

When examining an organization's medical benefits package, look first at the existing structure of the program and how it is received by providers and employees. The questions that follow will help you to focus on specific information.

Research Questions about the Policy

- What are the retention costs of the present policy?

  Is this cost more than the normal 6 to 10 percent?
  If so, why?
  Are these costs buried in administrative fees?

- If you are self-insured, what are your actual administrative costs?

  Are they more than 6 to 10 percent?
  If so, why?
  What will be necessary to reduce these costs?

- Is your benefits contract community-rated or experience-rated?

  If it is community-rated, as are most HMO plans, how can you determine the actual costs for your own employees?
  What effect will this rating have on efforts to control costs?
  What is your present loss ratio as determined by the paid basis report?
  How does the present loss ratio compare to the loss ratios of the last 3 years?

- How much is spent to cover claims? How does this compare with the total premium? Can the carrier explain discrepancies?

  Do you know how much is being spent on specific procedures by your group and how this compares with amounts spent in the previous 3 years?

- What trend figure is your carrier quoting?

- Are other employers in your area being quoted the same trend figure? Is your area one in which medical costs are higher or lower than average?

Research Questions about Your Employees

- Are your employees aware of the increasing problems with medical benefits and medical practices?

Decision Questions

- What approaches have been presented to you by your carrier or consultant on ways to reduce benefits costs?
- Can any of these suggestions be implemented within your company?
- Are you willing to commit the time and funds necessary to implement these changes?
- What programs can be initiated within your company to make employees aware of the growing problem of benefits costs?
- Which staff should be made available to disseminate this information?
- What groups, associations, or labor leaders need to be included in the effort to control costs?

Consumer Concerns

- Is my primary care physician a part of an HMO, PPO, or EPO? If so, is the structure of the organization preventing me from receiving the best care possible?
- Are my out-of-pocket expenses for medical care too high?
- Am I overusing my medical plan?
- Do I have a choice about which physician I see?
- Will my insurance plan allow me to see a specialist without first going through a primary care physician?

3
Becoming Part of the Solution

Everyone Is Part of the Problem and Should Be Part of the Solution

The Kaizen management theory speaks of the need to work toward continuous improvement of the organization through full participation. This theory can be applied successfully to design of an effective health benefits program. Cost-containment strategies can be rendered useless if those involved are not first brought into the process. Employers and employees, as well as brokers, consultants, health care providers, and insurance carriers must all work together to effect positive changes.

A Three-Phase Plan to Control Rising Medical Benefits Costs

In the current state of rising health care costs, a three-phase plan which capitalizes on the participation of every group within an organization to find solutions to the problem is essential. The first phase is covered in this chapter. Phase 2 is discussed in Chapters 4 and 5. The final implementation phase is detailed in Chapters 6 and 7. The three phases are:

Phase 1: Examination. Phase 1 focuses on an examination of the current state of the benefits program and the initiation of changes intended to keep the program solvent.

Phase 2: Evaluation.   In phase 2, a closer evaluation of the current benefits plan, the present carrier, and future needs and expectations is conducted.

Phase 3: Implementation.   The final phase of the plan includes implementation of a carefully developed plan designed to bring stability to the benefits program and to control current and future costs.

Full Participation Is Critical

Representatives from all sectors of the organization must be involved from the beginning. Managers are responsible for developing opportunities and mechanisms to enable all employee groups to get involved. The groups must work together to first understand the problem, then develop solutions. This process begins with the CEO and senior staff within the organization. Without the senior level of support, there will be no empowerment of those within the organization who are striving to effect a plausible solution.

Further, involvement must include educating the entire organization about the complexities of the medical care crisis as well as defining the problem nationally, locally, and in terms of the organization itself. Once employees have achieved this level of understanding, it is possible to move forward and to set goals for the organization. Alternatives and possible solutions can be developed and presented to brokers, consultants, and providers.

How to Establish an Insurance Committee

One effective method of involvement is to establish an insurance committee within your organization. A number of ways in which this can be accomplished are discussed below.

Committees in Small Organizations

If your organization has fewer than 4000 employees who are housed in close proximity, a single insurance committee can be formed. This committee would include representatives from top and middle management as well as all employee groups. If unions or negotiating groups are a part of your organization, they should be asked to provide two or three representatives to serve on the insurance committee. Ideally, these representatives should include the presidents or officers of those associations as well as rank-and-file members. Some senior staff members may initially be uncomfortable with this arrangement. However, the potential for serious, disruptive labor disputes centering on the issue of employee medical benefits should encourage even the most reticent executive to create a representative team of management and staff. This problem will only be solved through cooperation and trust.

Although, in some cases, committees with more than 8 members tend to become bogged down in personalities, in this situation a larger committee has been demonstrated to be effective. In fact, a general oversight committee as large as 25 people can be formed, with subcommittees for specific tasks.

Committees in Large Organizations

If an organization has more than 4000 employees or maintains several work sites over a large geographic area, it is more effective to form a committee at each work site. The work-site committees then elect several representatives to meet as an oversight committee. Figure 3-1 presents a sample agenda for an early meeting of the oversight committee. This agenda lays the groundwork for a beginning committee. In addition to committee members, the CEO or senior staff members should be present.

Senior Support for Committee Functions

Regardless of the size and configuration of the insurance committee, it must have visible senior support. The CEO should make frequent visits to the committee. Additionally, other senior management officials should be actively involved in working with the oversight committee as well as participating in some of the subgroup investigations and study sessions. Committee leadership should come from someone in the human resources or benefits management area. However, this leadership role should not include the power to make summary decisions or reversals of committee suggestions. The committee must function on a consensus basis; it must have power to make recommendations that will be utilized.

Many committees find it appropriate to spend the first sessions developing consensus and team-building skills, and becoming acquainted with one another. Once the members of the committee have established a working relationship with one another, they may then move toward establishing operating principles and setting long-term goals.

**Agenda
McWilliams and Farmer, P.C.
Insurance Committee**

1. Introduction of committee members and guests.
   Dave Farmer, *President*

2. General introduction; setting of ground rules for meeting.
   Gail Elmore, *Benefits Manager*

3. Introduction of Fred Briggs, consultant hired to work with committee.
   Bill McWilliams, *Vice President, Human Resources Division*

4. Statement of purpose.
   Bill McWilliams

Topics for Committee Discussion and Involvement

5. Open airing of immediate employee concerns or issues regarding benefits. (Comments welcome from all committee members. Gail Elmore will record concerns for consideration at future meetings.)
   - Listing of concerns
   - Selection of topics for future meetings

6. Operating agreements for future meetings. (Dave Farmer will chair.)
   - Committee goals
   - The decision-making process

7. Housekeeping items for future meetings. (Gail Elmore will chair.)
   - Dates, times, and places
   - Committee membership

Figure 3-1. Insurance committee agenda.

As the agenda illustrates, the first phase of the cost-containment process focuses on (1) organizing a committee drawn from all sectors of the company and (2) assisting committee members to establish a clear focus and a common goal. The goals for a company that is facing a benefits crisis will be quite different from those of a company that is analyzing and monitoring the current benefits program in an effort to avoid a crisis. Despite the differences in the present situation, both types of organizations will benefit from the three-phase approach to containing health benefits. Perhaps most important, a mechanism for ongoing analysis, input, and revision will be in place.

The Role and Responsibility of the Committee

One way of clarifying the committee's work is to focus on the three phases outlined previously. This process will require several months or more of study, implementation, and evaluation, followed by ongoing monitoring. These phases could include data gathering and implementation of short-term plan design changes, if needed, to stem large premium increases; analyses of data and restructuring of plan administration or design; and rebidding and implementation of a new plan if necessary. Even if substantive changes do not need to be made, it is important that the committee continue to gather and analyze data. Should the need to make changes arise, the mechanisms for effectively making those changes will be already in place. The committee chairperson should present this concept to all the members during an initial work session. An early understanding of the company's investment of time and money in an effort to control benefits costs often increases the members' level of commitment to success and alleviates fears that changes will be made too rapidly and without enough forethought or input.

Committee Guidelines

Following are some guidelines that should be used by the committee:

Representative membership. The committee must be representative of all groups in the organization and should include whoever is responsible for collective bargaining agreements or benefits and compensation.

Meeting times. If at all possible, the committee should meet on company time. Meeting on company time underscores the importance of the committee not only to its members but also to the whole organization. When meeting on company time is not possible because of varying work sites and shifts, a time which is convenient for the majority of committee members should be arranged. This meeting time should be chosen by the committee membership, not by the senior staff of the company.

Length of meetings. If necessary, hold one or two full-day meetings during which members analyze all the available data and the options resulting from that data. If the committee meets frequently enough, typically once a month, and if the meetings are well planned, then no more than three full-day meetings should be necessary over an 18-month period. The first full-day meeting should be devoted to examining the data and understanding the effects of the current plan design upon costs. Optional plan designs can be explored if necessary. Another day may be spent interviewing carriers, and a third deciding which carrier to select, if the committee's recommendations result in a rebidding of the company's medical and dental policies. If not, these additional meetings can focus on further analysis and examination of options.

Committee Education

Prior to dealing with specific data regarding the company medical and dental program, however, it is essential that the committee be educated on the subject of the medical care crisis in this country. In order to accomplish this, committee members must be supplied with information and time to spend reading, reviewing, and summarizing it. As part of the education process, it is useful to make available for review plan designs and premium costs of similar organizations in the area. These data are typically available through the broker or consultant with whom the company works, from local consultants who are seeking new clients, or from within the organization itself. These costs and plan designs should also be examined in light of national norms.

In order to accomplish their task effectively, committee members will have to develop a working vocabulary related to benefits programs. They will need to understand concepts such as *deductibles, copays, stop-loss, coinsurance,* and *maximum medical lifetime,* as well as common coverage terms such as *mental nervous disorder, speech therapy, subluxation,* and *major medical coverage.* These and other terms related to health care benefits are defined throughout this book and in the glossary.

The First Phase: Data Gathering

Once committee members have an overview of the national perspective—that is, once they understand the plan design and costs of their insurance program as compared with others in the area and in the nation—they may undertake an in-depth evaluation of the condition of their present plan. It is at this point that an outside consultant can be most helpful if an organization does not have a benefits person who can easily interpret the utilization data supplied by the carrier, the third party administrator, or the claims office.

Data the Committee Will Want to Examine

Information that the committee will want to examine includes the number of outpatient visits by type (CPT4s) and the total amount spent on these over a 3- to 5-year period by company employees. This data will make it relatively easy to project future outpatient costs provided there are no major changes in the plan design. Hospital admissions by type and length of stay should also be examined for that same 3- to 5-year period with careful consideration given to the total cost of the hospital stays and the increase in ambulatory or outpatient surgery. In addition, specific plan design provisions should be looked at in terms of their costs over the same period of time. For example, the frequency of inpatient and outpatient mental nervous disorder treatment should be analyzed.

This information should be available through your consultant, broker, or current carrier. Much of this information can also be found in larger local libraries. If data are not available for a 3- to 5-year period, start with what you do have and compare it to national and local norms. While there are thousands of procedure codes in the CPT4, the majority of claims tend to fall into fewer than 100 procedure categories. Work with your consultant to identify and compare the data you do have with the national norms for these codes.

How the Committee Can Acquire Employee Input

Phase 1 involves gathering initial data, setting goals, and making minor changes in the current plan, if necessary. Information on benefits needs should be gathered from every employee during this period. This should be done through an anonymous survey which allows employees confidentiality and the ability to state their needs without fear of reprisals.

Devising a Questionnaire

When devising this instrument, avoid canned questionnaires. The questions you use must reflect your organization and its employees' specific needs and concerns. The questionnaire should be short and yet contain enough statistical and geographical information to provide the committee and the consultant with enough information upon which to base decisions. An outside consultant should assist in development of the questionnaire. Ideally, the consultant should not be from the company's insurance carrier and should not represent other insurance companies.

Testing the Validity of the Questionnaire

Once the questionnaire has been developed, it should be tested on the committee members and randomly selected employees. Since committee members will already have a higher level of understanding of the problem, avoid using the committee as an exclusive sample. One of the major goals of this questionnaire is to find out what types of coverage are most essential to employees—even coverage that is not currently offered. It should also be determined what amount of money employees are willing to commit from their personal earnings to health care. This information should be compared with their current salaries, providing you with one measure of the importance of health care benefits in your employees' lives. The questionnaire should also contain a list of both satisfactions and dissatisfactions with the current program. Space can be provided for individual comments. While these can be difficult to tabulate, providing this space can be important to employee involvement. If the questionnaire is structured correctly, you will find that few employees avail themselves of the opportunity to write comments.

The Importance of Creating a Readable Questionnaire

The questionnaire should be printed in such a way as to make it easily understood by most employees. Ideally, employees should be given time during the day to preview the document and then answer the questions. However, if that is not possible, it should be distributed to each employee and collected within two days. While no employee's name need appear on the questionnaire, and every effort should be made to retain anonymity, it is important that some method be devised for ensuring that employees respond to the survey. In this matter, the committee can be helpful. Committee members can use their formal positions as well as their informal associations within the company to encourage employees to respond to the survey and to explain how it will be used.

If employees understand that the needs they express in that survey will be heard, the committee can expect a return rate of approximately 80 to 85 percent. A questionnaire developed using these guidelines is shown in Appendix B. This questionnaire enabled the group that used it to redesign its plan with committee and employee support, including reduction of some benefits and expansion of others.

Analyzing Data from the Questionnaire

Once the questionnaires have been collected, the data must be analyzed. The analysis should include cross-referencing of questions so that the conclusions will truly reflect the questionnaire results. In addition, the information should be analyzed with reference to all the other data gathered from the carrier in examination of the costs over a 3- to 5-year period. Based on this, the committee can then develop benefits goals for the organization.

Once the committee has defined the parameters of the program to be developed, the members should begin to work with the present carrier and the providers to determine their ability to meet the objectives of the program design and the needs of employees. If immediate changes are required to control escalating costs, it is at this point that those changes should be examined, evaluated, and initiated.

If the employee survey reveals major dissatisfaction with the present plan, and it thus becomes obvious that a major redesign of the benefits program is required, lines of communication between area providers, various carriers, and the committee should be established.

Initial Changes in Plan Design

While examining the figures for the previous 3 to 5 years, the committee will also wish to determine whether there were unusual trends or increases in costs. All the data collected should be compared with national and local norms. Armed with the data collected and the comparison data, the committee can understand fairly easily how premiums are and should be priced. The committee can then determine whether the organization's present plan design fits with its guidelines.

Organizations Using HMOs May Face a Problem in Acquiring Needed Information

Companies or organizations that use federally qualified HMOs will not have access to information that specifically addresses their employees.

They will need to research employee utilization using a survey instrument developed in-house, and will also need to work with the carrier to determine whether data specific to similar organizations can be obtained. The question is whether employees are actually spending more for health care than they pay in premiums.

Avoiding Pitfalls Created by Mandated Health Care

As committee members begin to question the data or individual costs within the plan, it is prudent to review federal regulations and mandated health care provisions. Because of mandated health care, some of the plan design changes the committee may propose cannot be implemented. Rather than meeting the frustration of trying to make changes which are subsequently disallowed, it is a better use of time to have committee members first research the parameters of mandated health care, thus avoiding potential pitfalls.

Although mandated health care legislation does affect the broad scope of a benefits plan, it is still possible to place controls on how those mandated benefits are utilized. Colorado, for example, has mandated that chiropractic services be included in any benefits program. As a result, it would be impossible for a company to redesign a plan without chiropractic benefits. However, the plan redesign can limit the number of visits to a chiropractor and the amount of money that would be reimbursed for each visit.

Moving toward Phases 2 and 3

Phase 2: Analyses and Assessment of the Current Situation

This immediate evaluation of the current situation leads directly into phase 2 of the committee's responsibilities, discussed in subsequent chapters. During this period, an in-depth analysis of costs and trends, as well as an assessment of the management capabilities of the insurance vendors, is conducted. Committee members should be concerned not only about the company's current insurance vendor or third-party administrator (TPA) but also about competing insurance companies and administrators.

Committee members should keep in mind that their responsibility is not necessarily to find a new carrier or TPA but to evaluate all available carriers and TPAs and select the best one for the company. The selection may, in fact, be the present carrier or TPA. Members should examine contracts, services, and the vendors' management structure and capabilities, and should also investigate ways in which the proposed program can be modified after a contract has been signed. This information, taken as a whole, will provide the company with a reference point for making decisions, and the company in turn will inform the committee of the various types of management strategies that are available.

Phase 3: Building a New Plan Design

Phase 3 involves competitive bidding for the medical and dental plan if it is deemed necessary to change carriers or plans. This is also the point at which strategic options should be developed for future planning. These strategic options will provide the committee and the company with ongoing information and data to use in meeting the needs of employees and any changes that may be brought about through legislation short of federally mandated health care.

Summary: Becoming Part of the Solution

The task of containing benefits costs is formidable yet not insurmountable. It is not a task to be completed by senior staff, insurance consultants, or TPAs alone. Any attempt at containing employee benefits costs must include employees. Formation of an insurance committee empowered to evaluate the present program and make any necessary changes has proved effective.

Membership of the insurance committee must include senior staff, employee associations and unions, and employees. Leaving any group unrepresented can seriously jeopardize the best efforts of the committee. Committee members must be willing to make an initial commitment of more than a year to the project. While it is possible for members to rotate on and off the committee, there should be a stable mix of old and new members at all times so that the education process will not need to be repeated.

There are no quick fixes available. In fact, for the efforts of the committee to be cost-effective, it is important that the committee remain in place even after a plan has been designed, implemented, and stabilized.

Without ongoing monitoring and evaluation, premiums can easily spiral out of control.

It is useful to look at the function of the committee as being made up of three distinct phases. During phase 1, the committee learns about the problem of rising medical health care costs, increasing attempts at legislating the problem, and the role each person might play in solving the problem.

During phase 1 the insurance committee should collect information from employees about their perceived health insurance needs. This information should be collected through an anonymous survey completed during work time if possible. The data collected from this survey are then analyzed to determine whether the present program is meeting employees' needs. If it is not meeting them, changes should be enacted if possible. Phases 2 and 3, which include further analysis of data and any needed plan design restructuring, are covered in subsequent chapters.

When changes have been effected in any phase of the process, every employee should receive information about the changes through company newsletters. Ideally, a benefits newsletter should be developed so that the minutes of committee meetings and summaries of the data can be made available to all members of the organization. Without this additional line of communication, it is possible to have a relatively informed committee making excellent decisions and then have to re-create the entire education process so that everyone within the organization will understand the changes. An even more disastrous situation can occur. If other members of the staff are not informed of the decisions made on their behalf, they may sabotage the work of the committee. Committee members can play a central role in employee education by reporting back to their respective associations and job sites after committee meetings, and by taking time at meetings to review what is happening and to delineate the reasons for those changes. It is a definite advantage to have this information disseminated as quickly as possible.

Focus Guide

Research Questions about the Current Program

- What is the current status of your medical benefits policy?

  Is it up for renewal soon?

  Have you received information from the carrier regarding proposed increases?

Research Questions about Your Employees and the Current Program

- Is there widespread dissatisfaction with the present program?

- Is the program experiencing overutilization?

- Is the question of medical benefits part of negotiations with employee groups?

Decision Questions about the Insurance Committee

- Whom will you charge with forming the insurance committee?

- Given the physical structure of the organization, will it be possible to have one insurance committee, or will it be necessary to form satellite committees, each reporting to an executive insurance committee?

- What steps will be taken to ensure complete participation throughout the organization?

- When and where will the committee meet?

Decision Questions about the Data-Gathering Process

- What steps will you take to assure that the committee has all the data it needs to review the present situation?

- Have you made your insurance consultant, broker, and carrier aware of the need for cooperation with the committee?

- Have you taken steps to adequately educate the members of the committee about the data they will review?

Decision Questions about the Questionnaire

- Is there someone within the committee structure who has the writing skills necessary to adequately write the questionnaire you will administer to employees?

- Has the questionnaire been adequately proofread and field-tested before being sent to the printer?

- Are all line managers and supervisors aware of the importance of the questionnaire? Has time been provided to allow for successful completion of the questionnaire?

- Have you set in place a process for reviewing the completed questionnaires and categorizing the data so that they can be reviewed by the insurance committee?

Consumer Concerns

- Can I be assured that my medical benefits will remain in force through this period of study by my employer's insurance committee?
- My utilization of the medical program has not been excessive, yet each year the amount of money I must contribute to my benefits increases. Why should I be responsible for these increases?

4

Getting Help: The Role of the Consultant

Insurance Consultants

All successful business strategies benefit from careful planning and a clear understanding of the situation at hand. The same elements are essential in evaluating a company's present and future medical benefits program. Since it is unlikely that senior staff members have the expertise necessary to successfully guide the company through the period of study and negotiation, it is advantageous to secure the services of an insurance consultant. The question is, what type of consultant will be most useful in bringing health care costs under control and devising a program to manage those costs once they have been controlled?

The Best Type of Consultant for Your Organization

Which type of consultant is best for an organization may be determined by studying the various types of consultants available to employers. Even if a company has already retained the services of a consultant, it is useful to periodically review the various types of consulting services available to determine whether the company is receiving the best help available.

When examining the various types of outside assistance available, one large employer was able to break consulting services down into three primary categories of service, described below. This rough division of services is not intended to delineate every service available from a consultant, but it can help an employer to focus on the primary services needed for a particular situation.

Broker-Consultants

Broker-consultants typically work for national firms that provide consulting and actuarial services. Many consulting firms maintain offices throughout the United States and bring a national perspective to their interpretation of a company's insurance situation.

Services Provided by Broker-Consultants. Broker-consultants are recognized as being extremely knowledgeable and having a good sense of the market. They use their expertise to the advantage of their clients by analyzing master contracts, suggesting needed changes to the plan design, assisting in the implementation of state and federal regulations, acting as negotiators with insurance carriers when necessary, and assisting in bidding for new contracts. In addition, some broker-consultants can also provide TPA services for companies wishing to design a self-insured program.

Broker-Consultants and Their Relationships with Carriers. Because broker-consultants work for large companies, they typically maintain close, positive relationships with insurance carriers. These carriers often are receptive to working with broker-consultants because they recognize that present and future contracts can be positively influenced through cooperation. Such close working relationships have the potential to interfere with the services provided by the consultant. For example, employers wishing to custom-design a plan or make modifications to a plan during the bidding process may find that the broker-consultant is reluctant to help since these changes may place a strain on a carrier with whom they work frequently. The employer is often willing to overlook this, because the value of the technical services provided by the consultant far outweighs the negative impact of the consultant's reluctance.

Paying for Broker-Consultant Services. Broker-consultants may be paid for their services in a variety of ways. Many are placed on an annual retainer, and others are paid a fee for service. Some consulting firms prefer to be paid a percentage of the plan they design for the client, typically between 1 and 5 percent of the annual premium. This fee is built into the policy's annual retention, and the insurance carrier reimburses the consultant directly. A consultant who assists a company in designing a fully self-insured program can be reimbursed through any of these same methods.

While the knowledge and expertise of a broker-consultant can be valuable, it is important to remember that such a consultant can be working for three employers: the consulting firm, the insurance carrier, and the company that has retained the consultant's services. Even if broker-consultants have no fee arrangements with carriers, it is important that they maintain good relationships with carriers for future work. While this situation in and of itself is not suspect, it should serve as a warning that the consultant may not be able to provide all the services that you need with as much objectivity as you want. Rely on the consultant particularly for technical backup, not complete plan design. Appendix A presents a letter of understanding from a large consulting firm to one of its clients.

Independent Consultants

Many employers turn to a second type of consultant to handle plan design and other specialized insurance-related services. Unlike the broker-consultant, the independent consultant is usually affiliated with a smaller firm that does not maintain offices throughout the country. Depending on the size of the independent consulting firm, employers can obtain the same services as described above.

Services Provided by Independent Consultants. When you retain an independent consultant, you should remember that such firms are small and often maintain only one office. They may not be able to provide as much technical backup in interpretation of federal and state regulations as larger consultants do. In spite of this limitation, they can still provide such services as TPA and bidding sources. In fact, these smaller firms are often more willing to tailor a program to a client's individual needs and to provide continuing support throughout the bidding process than are the larger firms. This willingness is vitally important if changes to the plan design are required during the bidding process.

While these small independent consultants often are flexible in their approach to plan design, they are not without their limitations. If the client is a large corporation with several thousand employees, it may be difficult for the independent consultant, working with a staff of four or five employees, to provide adequate support. Further, independent consultants are subject to influences within their own community such as local carrier and physician networks which limit the breadth of their perspective.

Paleo-Plan Plastics: The Unexpected Costs
of Rapid Growth in the Marketplace

Paleo-Plan Plastics had used the same insurance carrier for the past
decade. During those years, Paleo was a small company with several
dozen employees. The cost of insurance benefits continued to rise,
but there was no real concern about the situation. Two years ago
Paleo landed a lucrative contract to build packaging inserts for a
Japanese audio company. The work force at Paleo tripled in less
than a year, and insurance benefit costs began to skyrocket.

The CEO of Paleo turned to an insurance consultant for help in
controlling the costs. The local independent consultant assured
Paleo that a full range of consulting services was available, and that
after examining Paleo's master contract, provisions could be made to
bring costs under control.

After several weeks, the consultant recommended that Paleo
switch from a fully insured to a self-insured medical benefits
program. The consultant indicated that his firm was in a position to
provide TPA services. While the TPA services of this independent
consultant were excellent, Paleo felt that, given the company's
emerging international market, there were other issues to be
considered aside from plan administration. When the independent
consultant was asked to address this broader scope of issues, the
company discovered that the needed services could not be provided.
Paleo-Plan Plastics had inadvertently wasted several weeks and
thousands of dollars by selecting the wrong consultant.

The preceding example illustrates the need to determine what services a consultant can provide prior to establishing a working relationship with that consultant. Independent consultants who provide TPA
services often are likely to steer their clients toward self-insured programs requiring a TPA, since those TPA services provide the greater
portion of the consultant's income. While this arrangement is fine for
many companies, it is not the best for all.

Self-Employed Independent Consultants

Companies wishing to use an independent consultant but not interested
in TPA services can turn to either a self-employed independent consultant or an independent consultant working with a large independent
consulting firm.

Services Provided by Self-Employed Independent Consultants. The
primary function of the self-employed independent consultant is to

help the client understand the client's particular insurance problems and to broadly define available solutions. Some independent consultants have as their primary function the analysis of current insurance plans including program effectiveness and cost efficiency. Based on the findings, they are then able to make recommendations for improving the present plan design and administration.

Many of these self-employed independent consultants began their careers in large national broker consultant firms. As a result they often have a working relationship with both insurance carriers and TPAs. Because they are small and independent, potential clients should carefully evaluate consultants' references and work experience before contracting for service. Potential clients will want to determine the consultant's success at providing the specific services required. Since independent consultants' income is dependent solely from their ability to provide sound advice, their client bases will naturally grow as the number of organizations they have helped to control costs increases. You should discuss a consultant's services with one or more existing clients before retaining his or her services.

An independent consultant who works with a large independent consulting firm performs most or all of the services supplied by the other independent consultants, with one notable addition. Many independents are in a position to sell flexible spending accounts and related services. As is the case with the consultant who provides TPA services, this consultant may bring certain biases into the evaluation of a client's existing program. For example, if a client decides to institute flexible spending accounts (FSAs), the consultant may move the plan design toward services that can be provided at added cost by the consultant.

Independent consultants, whether they work alone, in small organizations, or in large independent firms, can assist clients in understanding problems and analyzing data. They are able to interface with carriers and large national consultants. Because their livelihood depends on service to the client, they are usually eager to provide quality service. The most successful independent consultants are as knowledgeable as those in the large insurance companies and consulting firms.

Insurance Carrier Representatives

Some employers may find that their current insurance carrier is in a position to offer consulting services. Because the services provided by carrier consultants cannot be without bias, their services should not be considered by a client wishing to examine options which extend beyond the scope of the current medical benefits plan or carrier. Rather than looking upon carrier representatives as consultants, it is wise to regard them as partners in controlling and managing the health care plan. This partnership is discussed in future chapters.

The Cost Benefit of Hiring a Consultant

In deciding which type of consultant to retain, cost must be a serious consideration. However, a small operating budget should never be regarded as a mandate to retain a consultant who receives fees from the insurance carrier. In the long run it is often more cost-effective to use a small independent consultant or one of the national consulting firms to analyze the present program. The needed savings can be realized through changes in plan design and administration over a period of time.

Templeton School District: Outside Consulting Services Reduce Overall Benefits Costs

When the Templeton Unified School District realized that its current medical benefits plan covering 2500 staff members was costing more money than the operating budget could afford, it turned to the insurance carrier for help. The carrier sent two representatives to work with the district's human resource manager. The advice these representatives provided seemed to address some of the short-run problems but fell far short of eliminating the problem.

Rather than accepting the plan changes prescribed by the company, the district retained the services of an independent consultant who billed the district on a fee-for-service basis. Although the consultant's expenses over 18 months exceeded $50,000, the changes he prescribed effected a $3 million savings in premiums and projected increases.

For most companies, it usually makes sense to retain either broker-consultants or local independent consultants who can provide TPA service and bidding sources. Such consultants can help you keep abreast of changing state and federal regulations, manage special projects such as COBRA implementation, or institute FSAs. They can also organize the bidding for new contracts and act as negotiators during premium renewal.

Whom to Hire and When

If the health care program of a company has experienced tremendous premium increases over the past few years, an independent consultant who provides no additional services should be retained to analyze costs and recommend changes. Retaining a small independent consultant will insulate the company from advice designed to increase the sale of related services rather than controlling costs. If it is not possible to engage the services of a small independent agent with strong references and an established record of success, the next best option is likely to be a large national consulting firm which can fully analyze the existing benefits program. Remain cognizant of existing biases and evaluate proposed plan changes in light of this reality.

Phased Analysis

As noted in the previous chapter, in order to maintain the greatest level of control over escalating costs, it is often useful to separate the analysis of the benefits program into three phases. Phase 1 examines the current state of the benefits program and initiates any immediate changes which must be made to keep the plan solvent. Phase 2 entails a closer evaluation of the current benefits plan, the carrier, and the future. Phase 3 marks the initiation of carefully developed plan design changes, if needed, which are designed to bring stability to the benefits program and control costs. Additionally, at this phase the development of future options as well as ongoing monitoring and evaluation take place. In each phase, an independent consultant should be asked to provide a list of the services that he or she can provide and what the cost to the client will be.

Marshall Bank and Trust: A Phased Approach to Controlling Medical Benefits Costs

During the past year, Marshall Bank and Trust (MB&T) had been engaged in a complete evaluation of its personnel services department. An analysis of the current health care benefits program was an integral part of this self-examination. For assistance in developing the best program possible for the dollars available, MB&T retained the services of a national insurance broker-consultant. Before bringing the consultant on board, MB&T senior staff had met to determine what function they wished the consultant to serve. They broke the insurance study into three phases: information gathering and analysis, immediate implementation of cost control measures if found necessary, and long-range planning.

This approach proved to be financially rewarding for MB&T. The savings realized from phase 1 was more than $156,000, representing actual dollar savings from reduced premiums. These funds were then applied to financing phase 2. Contracting for time-specific services on a relatively phase-specific basis enabled MB&T to control costs and to change the direction of the study when necessary.

The Cost of Consulting Services

Fee for Service

Clients often wrestle with the best method for paying for consulting services. Independent consultants who provide only advice and analysis are typically paid a fee for service. This financial arrangement works to the advantage of clients in that they are charged only for the services they need and are able to closely monitor the work being provided. While it may appear during some years that a retainer fee is more cost-effective, it is often more difficult to demand specific services from a consultant working on a retainer basis.

For example, one company with 3600 insureds was paying a national broker-consultant an annual retainer, which in the current year was approximately $16,000. This fee included any bidding service needed, and there was an annual renegotiation of the carrier's contract. In addition, information as needed was supplied to the company. However, in analyzing costs over a several-year period it became clear that there were many years during which few services were used with the exception of the annual review of premium increase. Obviously, the retainer arrangement was not in the best fiscal interest of the company.

Companies of moderate size will probably find it best to use a fee-for-service arrangement. Within that fee structure, additional services can be provided on either an hourly or a by-service basis, should the need arise. This arrangement allows the client to maintain firm control over the dollars being spent.

Fee-for-service agreements should be reviewed annually or biannually to allow for proper budgeting. At each renewal, the client should review the quality of services received from the consultant and determine whether each service provided should be continued. Some basic decisions about future client-consultant relations should be made prior to meeting with the consultant. During the meeting, the annual fee should also be renegotiated.

Specific services should be listed under the fee-for-service arrangement, and other services which might be needed should be noted, along with a specific price for each such service. This procedure should enable a client to budget for services required or anticipated.

Retainer

If an organization opts for a retainer fee, it is wise to request from the consultant a schedule of fees charged for specific services. This added information allows the client to assess whether the retainer is being overutilized or underutilized, and should be included in the annual review of the client-consultant relationship. National broker-consultant firms may prefer a retainer over a fee-for-service arrangement if they are not being paid a percentage of the premium directly from the carrier.

If this is the case, the client should ensure that expected services are listed in the agreement so that there will be no misunderstanding during the course of the contract. If the broker-consultant with whom the client contracts is paid by the carrier, the need for specifically listing the services to be provided by the consultant to the client becomes paramount. It is up to the client to determine whether this arrangement is cost-effective. The client should determine whether the services being provided are adequate for effectively monitoring costs and keeping them under control. If not, it would be advisable to retain an independent consultant to assist with the monitoring process.

Summary: Remaining Involved

Acquiring Consulting Services

The retention of consultant services does not alleviate a client's obligation to remain involved in controlling and managing the costs of the company's medical benefits program. It is not wise management strategy to hire a large national broker-consultant firm and turn the entire insurance program over to it. This approach would prove extremely costly, not only in accumulating fees for service or retainer arrangements but also in the type of program designed for the company. Do not expect a consulting firm to customize health care packages for clients not willing to become involved in working to achieve the desired outcomes. A company that does not work closely with its consulting firm is likely to receive a standardized benefit plan that may not meet the specific needs of the company or its employees.

The same caveat applies to the hiring of independent consultants. An independent consultant who has been hired to evaluate an existing program, cannot complete the job without company involvement. If possible, one or two staff members should be assigned to work with the independent consultant on an ongoing basis to monitor time lines and recommendations. Experienced consultants demand cooperation and assistance from the organization they are serving. Only through close communication can a plan be adequately analyzed and recommendations developed which are tailor-made to the organization. If an organization is not willing to invest time, its ability to manage its benefits plan from a cost-containment perspective will be compromised.

Consultants and the Insurance Committee

Finally, whatever type of consultant is selected, the understanding should be that one of his or her primary responsibilities is to meet on a regular basis with the organization's insurance committee. In the beginning, there will be a need for frequent meetings with the consultant to educate the committee members about the committee's purpose and goals, to respond to their questions, and to gather data and present analyses. Once these functions have been fulfilled, usually after 12 to 18 months, fewer meetings will be required. For example, if a large national broker-consultant firm has been retained, not only should representatives of this firm be attending all the company's committee meetings but also they should be in a position to provide committee members with information on pertinent federal and state legislation and regulations, a review of plan design and cost, and an analysis of similar plans in the geographic area. Further, the consultants should meet with the committee on a quarterly basis to respond to questions and to review utilization data.

If an organization chooses to use the services of an independent broker-consultant, it should be made clear at the beginning of the relationship what meetings and what information will be needed during the initial and succeeding phases. If the independent consultant does not have the resources to provide all the information needed, other methods of obtaining this information will need to be found.

Data Presentation

Whatever type of consultant is selected, the consultant should be prepared to present to committee members not only the data but also alternatives based on them, so that decisions can be based on fact and consensus. The consultant should assist in analysis of data and examination of options. Employers should remember that the consultant is retained to provide a service; if that service is not forthcoming in the anticipated manner, other consulting options should be explored. Working with consultants to examine data is covered in the next chapter.

Focus Guide

Research Questions about Your Organization's Consulting Needs

- What services are being provided by the current consultant?
- Is the organization depending too heavily on consulting services provided directly by the carrier?
- What services do you wish to have your consultant provide?

Decision Questions about Your Consultant

- Has the consultant retained by your organization agreed to work closely with your insurance committee?
- Has the consultant been able to secure the data your committee needs to make an educated decision about the future of the medical benefits program?
- Is the consultant hired by your organization in a position to work with your present carrier?

5
What Should Be Examined

Moving Forward

Simply recognizing that costs of medical care benefits are edging or soaring out of control will do nothing to alleviate the problem. Before any action designed to bring costs under control and to deliver more effective service to employees is taken, a thorough analysis of current costs and plan designs must be conducted. This study period represents the second phase of the insurance study.

Once fact finding has occurred, the organization's insurance committee, working with the consultant, can determine what, if any, changes should be made in the existing plan design. Using the data collected through the evaluation, the committee will be able to determine whether the current carrier or administrator of the medical plan is meeting the service needs of the organization. Whatever the determination, the analysis must be carried out in a thorough and thoughtful manner, for the effects on delivery of services to employees and on the cost of the plan will have far-reaching effects.

Initiation of Phase 2

During the second phase of the insurance study, the consultant should support the designated company representative by sharing the lead role in analyzing the data collected from employees, the carrier, and participating providers. While receiving the consultant's summary, committee members should remain cognizant of any biases the consultant may bring to the task. It is essential that all committee members have a work-

ing knowledge of the terminology, structure, and information presented in the reports they examine.

Types of Medical Coverage

The first area to be examined should be the type of medical coverage
currently offered to employees. Is the program fully insured or self-
insured? Each program has inherent advantages and disadvantages, including the cost risk assumed by the employer. Committee members
should be aware of the unique characteristics of each funding approach,
as well as the ramifications of each for the organization.

Fully Insured Programs

Fully insured programs are those in which the employer agrees to remit
a complete premium to a carrier and in return receive medical coverage
for all eligible employees and their covered dependents. Coverage is often in the form of a traditional indemnity program, which provides full
services to employees, with set deductibles, coinsurance, and stop losses.
Under fully insured indemnity programs an employee may select any
medical provider to perform needed services. Claims are then submitted to the carrier for payment.

Provider Options in a Fully Insured Program.   Fully insured programs
might also include a PPO or EPO option whereby employees would pay
less in coinsurance and deductibles if they obtained medical services
from a group of doctors selected by the insurance carrier for their willingness to provide services at set fees. A fully insured program might
also offer an HMO as an option.

Distinguishing Characteristics of a Fully Insured Program.   In a fully
insured program the company sends the full premium amount to the
carrier, which then becomes responsible for setting aside the necessary
funds from the premium for reserves and retention fees. At the end of
each contract period, the carrier negotiates any needed increases in the
premium to cover costs. The employer's responsibility under a fully insured plan is simply to write the check for the correct amount at the
correct time.

Community and Experience Ratings
in Fully Insured Programs

Under a fully insured program, there are two ways in which the program can be rated for premium consideration: it can be community-

rated or experience-rated. Under a fully insured community-rated program, the carrier determines the premium amount by looking at the utilization experience for all insureds in a geographical area who are covered under a particular plan design, whether or not they work for the same employer. Some community-rated programs may include everyone in a particular state who is covered under a specific plan design.

Advantages of a Community-Rated Program. The advantage of community rating is that a small employer with only 25 to 30 employees can spread the risk of a catastrophic illness striking an employee through a much larger group of individuals. Most HMOs are fully community-rated. The disadvantage of the community-rated program is that a specific employer cannot find out the medical costs of his or her particular employees, and thus cannot know how these costs are contributing to rising premiums. Conversely, if premiums become stabilized, the employer is unable to determine whether this is due to the other members of the community-rated pool or because the claims experience of his or her own employees is improving.

Fully insured programs can also be experience-rated. In this situation, the premium cost for the medical coverage is based solely on the experience of the employees covered under an employer's particular plan. Experience rating provides organizations with an incentive to keep costs under control as future premiums will be based on these costs. Experience rating is advantageous in that it allows the employer and the insurance committee to analyze the specific costs of their own program.

Advantages of an Experience-Rated Program. Experience rating may offer an employer some flexibility in making premium payments, as well. In some instances, fully insured programs that are experience-rated will allow an employer to pay the premium on a monthly basis. The advantage of this payment schedule is that the employer can make financial use of the total premium delay through short-term investments. In reality this becomes a partially insured program. But the delayed premium does not mean that the client is not responsible for the full amount of the premium. At renewal, premiums will increase if the combined loss ratio, retention, and needed reserve charges, along with trend, exceed the previous annual premium.

Self-Insured Programs

Just as there are several types of fully insured programs, an employer can also find several types of self-insured programs. Many people mistakenly believe that a self-insured program requires an employer to completely administer medical coverage in-house or through a TPA, and to fully fund all medical expenses, with an optional stop-loss policy should there be a catastrophic claim. While this is one possible design, it is only one of three commonly implemented approaches.

Contracting for Services with a Self-Insured Program.   A partially self-insured plan enables the employer to pay a minimum premium and hold the reserves internally, and also to collect the interest accruing from reserves. Under this type of self-insured program, an employer can contract with a carrier to provide a specific coverage such as a traditional indemnity, a PPO, an EPO, an HMO, or any effective combination. In turn, the employer pays a minimum premium to the carrier and maintains three benefits accounts: one for retention, one for medical claims, and a third for reserves. Each of these accounts is funded separately. Usually the company pays the carrier a monthly minimum premium and retention fee.

Funding Arrangements.   Many employers are unaware that in a partly self-insured program they can hold the interest, using the income for any variety of purposes. When examining a self-insured program, an employer will be wise to determine who will receive the interest under the funding agreement, rewriting that agreement if necessary. The self-insured minimum premium program looks much like a fully insured program. The primary difference is in the employer's level of liability. The carrier who is delivering services under this plan can pay for a stop-loss policy for the company, to cover any claims which exceed a certain amount, typically $80,000 to $100,000. These stop-loss provisions serve to reduce the risk of any program. However, under a self-insured program, a company can decide to forgo the stop-loss policy if its reserve is high enough to cover a catastrophic claim. As with fully insured programs, the following year's premiums will depend upon the experience of the group as well as the amount needed to cover retention, reserves, and trend. Table 5-1 details the characteristics of the various forms of insurance.

Third-Party Administration.   When using a fully self-insured program, an employer can contract with a third-party administrator (TPA) to pay claims and purchase stop-loss coverage. The employer holds the reserves and pays the administrator for the incurred medical expenses plus any administrative costs. Since employees submit their claims directly to the TPA, the employer should expect to incur regular administrative costs under this program. These administrative costs typically range from 6 to 10 percent of premium payments, depending upon the type of stop-loss coverage provided and the type of reports the employer requests from the TPA.

Table 5-1. Forms of Insurance and Self-Insurance

Fully insured	Partially insured	Partially self-insured	Fully self-insured
Community-rated or pooled contract	Experience-rated contract	Minimum premium contract	Administrative or claims-services-only contract, or self-administration
Options	Options	Options	Options
Large deductibles or coinsurance	Retrospective premium agreement	Expected claim level selection	Individual stop-loss policy
	Delayed-premium agreement	Unfunded reserve liability	Aggregate stop-loss policy

SOURCE: William T. Barnes Consulting.

In-House Administration.   In another type of fully self-insured program, the employer fully administers the medical benefits program in-house. Instead of paying administrative costs to a TPA or carrier, the employer hires the necessary personnel to process and pay claims and prepare reports. In addition, the employer can purchase a stop-loss policy to cover against catastrophic illness or any aggregate claims running over a specified amount.

All self-insured programs are essentially experience-rated since the cost of the program is determined only by the individuals enrolled in it. There has been a misconception that being self-insured will save an employer a substantial amount of money. This is not necessarily true, since all costs including administration, reserves, and medical claims must be paid. Some unwary employers have gotten themselves into trouble by not holding back enough reserves. Under this plan, a sudden increase in the number of submitted claims could have a damaging effect on a company's operating expenses.

The only effective method of saving money when working with medical benefits is through cost-containment strategies and careful review of expenses. Employers, whether self-insured or fully insured, that have experience-rated medical benefits programs and the proper reports can analyze the costs of their programs rather easily. Fully insured employers that use a community-rated program will find it more difficult to assess why premiums are increasing.

Risk Transference upon Termination

Expenses Incurred but Not Reported

After studying the insurance program in effect, the committee and consultant should analyze the risk-transference provisions that will go into effect upon termination of the policy. Every premium has built into it a cost for incurred but not reported (IBNR) claims. These claims are submitted following the end of a policy year for services rendered during the previous year. When a policy is terminated, it is expected that claims will continue to be received for at least 3 months and up to a year. Many carriers place a limitation upon the time that they will honor claims following termination. In addition, it is now common for the carrier to ask that the employer or policyholder be liable for a predetermined percentage of the IBNR claims at termination if the amount held in reserves is insufficient to cover the IBNR claims. In addition to the liability of IBNR claims which occurs at the start of each premium year (even if there is no termination), there are extension of benefit (EOB) provisions which must be addressed.

Extension of Benefits

Traditionally, most policies have an EOB provision which directs that, upon termination of the policy, any covered individual who is disabled and unable to perform his or her work will be covered for that disability only under the old policy for a specified period of time or until one of three events occurs:

- The person is able to return to active work or resume a normal schedule.
- The person has obtained coverage from another source.
- The period of coverage under the EOB provision has passed.

When evaluating the effectiveness of the medical benefits program, committee members will want to look at the dollar amount that the carrier or program administrator wishes to place into reserves to cover EOB. Normally 8 to 10 percent of the total reserve applies to EOB. However, if the EOB provision includes disabled retirees or individuals on long-term disability, the percentage will likely be greater. This increase can be avoided by writing the EOB provision to include only active employees who are disabled at the time of policy termination but who have not been placed on long-term disability or disability retirement. All other disabled individuals can be covered by the new plan.

Because individuals falling under the EOB provisions are critically ill or in need of extensive treatment, it is to the carrier's or plan administrator's advantage to carefully limit this provision through its definition of eligible participants. It is often to the employer's advantage to have a broad EOB provision so that upon termination and transition to a new carrier and/or policy, first-year costs can be relatively contained. Although EOB provisions do not go into effect until policy termination, the definitions agreed upon at the beginning of the policy or in succeeding years are those which will govern eligibility. To avoid potential problems, EOB definitions should be written carefully, and the meaning of those definitions should be clear to both the carrier and the employer. Even so, litigation can result if the carrier or plan administrator finds a loophole in the policy which will excuse the carrier from responsibility.

Maximum Termination Liability

Some carriers have begun to insist that the policyholder accept liability for all claims which exceed the reserves submitted following termination. For this reason and others, when contracting for medical benefits, an employer should carefully examine maximum termination liability (MTL). Under this provision, the carrier cannot ask the policyholder for additional funds following contract termination even if the IBNR and EOB claims exceed the reserves.

MTL places the entire risk of transference upon termination onto the carrier. Therefore, the carrier is holding a greater risk than it would prefer. Many carriers will provide an MTL clause only if the policyholder is willing to pay an additional percentage fee for this arrangement. If the percentage requested is more than 6 to 10 percent, the carrier should be closely questioned about why the percentage is so high. Before an employer elects to pay for MTL, he or she should determine whether the additional costs are warranted. A company may opt for minimum termination liability to reduce premiums or because it is counting on few IBNR and EOB claims. An employer that chooses this route should be aware of what it is getting in termination liability, and of the possible effects.

An employer who is aware of the true cost of the medical benefits program, and who has cost-containment measures in place, is in a strong position to negotiate an MTL clause with little or no increase in premiums. One caveat: review the reserve costs. Some carriers will agree to the MTL clause without an increase in premiums because they have shifted a greater percentage of the total premium into the reserve account, thereby reducing the amount available to pay medical claims and increasing the amount available for IBNR and EOB.

Central Mountain Bottling: Negative
Effects of Reduction in Work Force on
Medical Benefit Costs

Central Mountain Bottling (CMB), a large regional distributor for
three lines of soft drinks, had recently won several concessions from
its operating unions. CMB needed to significantly modernize its
four plants in order to remain competitive. Strategic planning called
for addition of five new fully automated bottling lines, which would
result in the loss of 75 labor and 3 clerical positions. In return for
this union concession, CMB management agreed, among other
things, to bolster the existing medical benefits program. The CEO
assigned the task of negotiating with the carrier to the assistant
director of personnel.

The employees who had least seniority were dismissed, and the
remaining employees began training for their new jobs in the
automated plant. CMB management had negotiated an improved
benefits plan with the existing insurance carrier. As part of the plan
redesign, the carrier agreed to add an MTL clause to the benefits
contract for a small increase of 3 percent of the total premium.

Initially, things seemed to be going smoothly. But they were not.
When the new benefits plan came up for annual review and
negotiation, the carrier demanded a 63 percent increase in
premium. When they analyzed the carrier's proposal, CMB officers
realized that they had not carefully evaluated their position when
negotiating the benefits contract. By laying off the employees with
less seniority, CMB had increased the average age of employees.
Older employees often require more medical attention, which drives
up utilization. Further, the carrier had diverted a higher percentage
of the premium into reserves to cover the MTL clause, thus
reducing the funds available to pay medical claims. These two
situations worked in concert to drive up premiums. CMB and its
insurance carrier must share the responsibility.

Retention Costs Written into
Premium Contracts

Another area that needs to be considered in the total medical benefits
program is the level of retention written into the contract. Retention
costs include applicable taxes; a risk charge for stop-loss coverage; any
expenses which may be incurred through use of a PPO, an HMO, or an
EPO; claims handling; and overhead. Retention may also include hid-
den charges such as commissions received by consultants from carriers.
As a general guide, retention costs should run from 6 to 10 percent of
the premium.

Table 5-2 provides an example of breakdown of retention charges for

Table 5-2. Renewal Action Statement
Retention (10/1/86 to 10/1/87)

Medical (Net Premium: $2,725,572)		
Taxes	$ 11,993	0.44%
Risk charge	27,256	1.00
PPO expense	33,600	1.23
Claims handling*	157,794	5.79
Interest credit	−35,432	−1.30
Administrative expense	55,542	2.04
Total	$ 250,753	9.20%
Dental (Net Premium: $550,595)		
Taxes	$ 1,376	0.25%
Risk charge	5,506	1.00
PPO expense		0.00
Claims handling†	27,132	4.93
Interest credit	−7,158	−1.30
Administrative expense	25,451	4.62
Total	$ 52,307	9.50%

*Drafts 24,276 @ $6.50.
†Drafts 5,712 @ $4.75.

a medical and dental program. An employer should carefully study the list of charges under its retention clause and closely question what is covered by each. Even with this documentation, it is possible for carriers to place other costs under administrative expense. Each cost should be carefully examined, and if the need arises, documentation should be requested.

Carriers' Margin

Carriers also prefer to add a carriers' margin, or claims fluctuation factor, to their policies. This percentage of total premium price may appear under retention or trend, or may be noted as a separate item. The claims fluctuation factor further insulates the carrier against loss. Given the current high trend factors, an employer should closely question the carrier plan administrator about the addition of margin.

Health Maintenance
Organizations

If the medical benefits program includes a health maintenance organization (HMO), additional factors must be examined. As noted earlier, most HMOs are community-rated; as a result, it is difficult to examine the true costs of the program and the actual amounts of money that employees are costing an individual employer.

Adverse Selection with HMOs

Another factor that can occur with HMOs is called *adverse selection*. If an HMO is offered side by side with a traditional indemnity program with high deductibles, it is likely that the healthier employees will select the HMO, while the less healthy employees will enroll in the indemnity plan. Because an individual cannot receive specialized services in an HMO without approval of an assigned doctor, less healthy individuals tend to select the indemnity programs, which allow them to use their own doctors and receive treatments at the hospitals of their choice rather than using HMO services.

When healthy employees select the HMO and the less healthy select a traditional indemnity program, adverse selection results. The cost of the traditional indemnity program skyrockets, and the employer is faced with rising premiums.

Advocates of HMOs argue that if adverse selection were truly an issue, it would be affecting them because they provide greater coverage at a lower price, thus attracting those consumers placing a high demand on medical services. This has not proved to be the case, however. Further, the HMO cost-cutting approach to medical services has resulted in a rash of HMO bankruptcies over the past few years, causing deterioration in some consumers' confidence in the ability of HMOs to meet their needs. Currently, the HMOs that have survived have often done so by raising rates.

Mandated HMO Services

HMO plans will continue to proliferate, however, as legislation allows federally qualified HMOs to mandate that an employer with 25 or more employees must add an HMO option to the medical benefits program, if one is not already in place. The mandate must be made 6 months prior to renewal of the employer's premium contract. This law will remain in effect until October 24, 1995.

Although a company that has been mandated to include an HMO option is required to comply with the mandate, it is not required to add the particular HMO that brought the action. What it must do, however, is add the same *type* of HMO in the same geographic location as the one which brought the action. Currently, there are three types of HMOs:

- HMOs that include a large number of doctors who are a part of an Independent Physicians Association (IPA) model
- HMOs that are part of a clinic (staff model)
- HMOs that are part of a large organization providing only HMO services (group model)

Mitigating the Problems Caused by Mandated HMO Plans

If an employer is mandated to add an HMO option to the medical benefits program, many problems can be mitigated by electing the HMO plan of the existing carrier, if it offers the type of HMO being mandated. This will allow the adverse selection to be spread across both plans. The HMO option should be priced as high as possible under governing regulations, to offset any adverse impact. Figure 5-1 provides a

---

1. What benefit plans are currently available to your employees? What options are available to individual subscribers? What is the current enrollment in each of these plan options? Does your company have any "new" plans with which it is experimenting for any employee group—active or retired?

2. What are the rates for your plans? How are these rates determined and how often are they evaluated? Are employer-specific rates such as age-step available?

3. How can you as an employer find out how the fair value of the services received by your employees (and/or their dependents) compares with the actual amount of premiums paid?

4. What data are your current HMO willing to share with you about the services used by a particular employee group?

5. What methods are available to determine the cost for these services on either an employer-specific or a community basis?

6. What steps must your employees take to be reimbursed for emergency services provided outside the contracted HMO service area? Indeed, *can* they be reimbursed for these expenses?

7. Is your present HMO financially stable? Is the HMO in a position to provide documentation that can adequately predict future financial stability? If the HMO is unable to provide this financial forecast, what steps has it taken to remain financially solvent?

Figure 5-1. HMO questions.

list of questions that employers can use to gather data on HMO programs.

Although most HMOs are currently community-rated, federally qualified HMOs are now able to provide a combination of community and experience ratings for employers. This allows employers who do offer HMOs to receive more data concerning their plan participants and to develop some control over the cost of the HMO premium. While the HMO approach to delivery of medical services appeals to many consumers, the premise that any benefit offered should have its costs reflected in the premium still exists. If employees are to receive first-dollar coverage for all treatment, the cost of that coverage should be considerably higher than the cost for coverage that does not include first-dollar coverage or that sets high deductibles and copays, as do many traditional indemnity programs.

Plan Design

A final step in evaluating the current benefits program is to carefully examine the plan design and the costs of the plan components. What is offered or covered can unwittingly drive costs up by encouraging people to use more. Several documents that should be available from the carrier or plan administrator can assist you in conducting a thorough and efficient review of the costs of the present plan. The case study which follows details one organization's progress through this process.

Stafford Farms: Analyzing the Cost of a Medical Benefits Plan

Background

Stafford Farms is a successful mail-order venture with headquarters in New England. Each year, millions of consumers purchase Stafford's exclusive line of clothing and accessories. To meet growing demand, Stafford Farms employs 2295 people and conducts ordering and shipping services 24 hours a day, 7 days a week, excluding national holidays.

One reason for Stafford Farms' continuing success is its comparatively relatively low markup on goods. Operating at a low profit margin requires Stafford's management team to watch operating expenses even more closely than do their competitors. When it became clear that rising insurance benefit costs were threatening to explode across the bottom line, Stafford's CEO directed the company's insurance committee to thoroughly examine the existing program. After examining the structure of the program, the committee requested specific cost figures from the current carrier. Working with the consultant, the committee examined current costs and made several decisions designed to bring costs under control.

First Steps: The Work of the Insurance Committee

The insurance committee first examined the gross breakdown of plan costs, as outlined in Tables 5-3 and 5-4. The monthly cost for medical claims was averaging $135 for each of the 2295 employees. However, utilization varied tremendously among the employees: 110 Stafford employees should have been paying $1490 a month for the amount of coverage they received, while the majority of insured should have only been paying $72. Table 5-4 displays the same information in a slightly different manner. It shows that 3 percent of Stafford's insureds incurred no costs and 83.5 percent of the insureds incurred less than $104 a month. While insurance is based on the premise that some individuals will need greater coverage than others, the monthly premium for Stafford Farms was $92—far less than the amount necessary to pay claims. Using the information drawn from the exhibits, it was clear to the insurance committee that the premium would have to rise more than 40 percent to cover claims alone. The carrier was demanding a 70 percent increase in premium to cover medical claims, build up its reserves, and offset against trend, then running at 25 percent.

Table 5-3. Stafford Farms, Inc.
Medical Plan Cost Breakdown, 1988

	Paid medical claims		Number of employees		Actual average annual cost per employee	Actual average monthly cost per employee
	$3,710,435	÷	2,295	=	$ 1,618	$ 135
Families incurring costs over $5,000	1,966,531	÷	110	=	17,878	1,490
Families incurring costs under $5,000	1,743,904	÷	2,028	=	860	72
Families incurring no costs	0	÷	157	=	0	0

Table 5-4. Stafford Farms, Inc.

Medical Plan Costs—Sample Distribution*

Annual benefits	Monthly cost	Number of employees and dependents	Percentage
$80,000–100,000	$7,500	2–3	0.1
60,000–79,999	5,833	3–5	0.2
50,000–59,999	4,583	4–7	0.2
40,000–49,999	3,750	5–8	0.3
30,000–39,999	2,916	6–10	0.3
20,000–29,999	2,083	10–15	0.5
10,000–19,999	1,250	20–25	1.0
5,000–9,999	625	60–90	3.3
2,500–4,999	312	150–200	7.6
0–2,499	104	1,500–1,800	83.5
0	0	150–200	3.0
Total: $3,700,000	$ 135	2,300	100.0

*Based on 1988 actual results.

Going into Detail: Using All Available Data

The gross breakdown of costs provided Stafford's insurance committee with only a portion of the picture. The information did not indicate whether there were specific plan design abuses or whether the increasing costs were due to inflated provider charges or to a few unusually expensive illnesses. Therefore, a more specific breakdown was needed. Table 5-5 shows the distribution of charges made against the plan from October 1, 1983, to October 1, 1987. It is clear that there were two areas in which plan costs had spiraled. Physician charges escalated from 11.8 percent of the total to 16.5 percent of the total in just 4 years, whereas the normal percentage of the total increase should have been 3.7 percent according to the carrier. Second, X-ray and lab charges increased to 9.9 percent from 6.3 percent, whereas the normal percentage of the total increase should have been 5.5 percent according to the carrier. In short, the normal percentage of the total increase should have been far less than was indicated by plan usage. Charges had increased over $1 million in just 4 years. Although the ratio of paid charges to claims had actually dropped, this decrease was attributable to increased premiums paid by Stafford Farms. Although the carrier was not losing money on the account during this period, Stafford was becoming strapped. The company could not afford to increase premium payments again to keep pace with increased usage.

A further examination of the physicians' charges indicated extremely

Table 5-5. Stafford Farms, Inc.
Distribution of Charges

	10/1/83 to 9/1/84		10/1/84 to 9/1/85		10/1/85 to 9/1/86		10/1/86 to 10/1/87		Normal
	Charges	% of total	Charges	% of total	Charges	% of total	Charges	% of total	% of total
Hospital	$ 963,186	45.7	$1,254,311	46.7	$ 940,697	36.7	$1,200,485	35.0	48.8
Room, bed	336,923	16.0	430,759	16.0	277,764	10.8	418,173	12.2	16.8
Inpatient, misc.	475,303	22.5	636,568	23.7	470,622	18.4	594,467	17.3	26.4
Outpatient, misc.	150,960	7.2	186,985	7.0	192,311	7.5	187,845	5.5	5.6
Surgical	292,633	13.9	363,377	13.5	386,840	15.1	456,517	13.3	14.2
Physician	248,326	11.8	322,764	12.0	366,009	14.3	567,086	16.5	3.7
X ray and lab	133,872	6.3	150,930	5.6	216,229	8.4	340,431	9.9	5.5
Other covered charges	470,729	22.3	595,183	22.2	654,485	25.5	869,803	25.3	27.8
Total charges	$2,108,746	100	$2,686,564	100	$2,564,260	100	$3,434,322	100	100
Total benefits	$1,786,817		$2,309,060		$2,067,780		$2,804,941		
Paid claims	1,610,772		2,079,173		2,065,343		2,607,995		
Paid/charge ratio		76.4		77.4		80.5		75.9	

high costs in the area of psychiatric and chiropractic usage. These costs are detailed in Table 5-6. More than $265,000 was spent for chiropractic charges alone from the period September 1, 1987, to September 1, 1988. This was equivalent to approximately one-tenth of the total cost of the plan on an annual basis. For the 6-month period from January 1, 1988, to June 1, 1988, the psychiatric benefits were running more than $109,000, or approximately 10 percent of the total plan cost. Clearly, this situation could not continue if Stafford was to continue providing employee medical benefits.

While it was clear that there was overuse on the part of employees, it also became clear that there had been a tremendous increase in the costs of the services. Table 5-7 indicates that paid claims increased more than $700,000 over a 2-year period. This increase could not be attributed to usage since the number of exposures or claims submitted decreased by 1600. The average cost of each claim, however, had increased by almost $30. Either there had been a tremendous increase in the costs of services or more complex services were now being provided.

In actuality, a combination of the two was occurring. Over a 3-year period the PPO network of doctors used by Stafford employees had increased their fees by 15 percent, whereas non-PPO doctors in the same area had increased their fees by only 7 percent as illustrated in Table 5-8.

The number of services used by staff had decreased 1 percent between 1987 and 1988, after a sharp increase between 1986 and 1987 of 19 percent, as detailed in Table 5-9.

The PPO Situation: Stafford's Loss of Control

The combination of a 15 percent increase in PPO fees in 1988 and a 1 percent decline in usage during the same period indicated that a phenomenon known as *code creep* was also taking place, coupled with an increase for each procedure. Claims for office visits were being coded as extended rather than routine. Code creep, while not severe in this case, combined with the increase in physicians' fees to contribute to the overall 15 percent increase.

Still to be resolved was why usage had increased so dramatically in 1987. While it had decreased 1 percent in 1988, it was still 18 percent over the 1986 usage figures. In 1986, on the advice of the carrier, Stafford Farms had instituted the PPO plan which featured a $5 patient copay for each office visit.

The intended purpose of the PPO option was to reduce costs by reducing the cost of medical service. Yet, the information presented in

Table 5-6. Stafford Farms, Inc.

Chiropractic Service Charges and Benefits

Services	Charges	Benefits
10,130	$367,375.59	$265,222.59

Professional Psychiatric Service Charges and Benefits

	Claims	Services	Charges	Benefits
Office	307	3,016	$209,535.12	$109,225.64
Inpatient	5	74	$8,834.00	$7,853.20

Table 5-7. Stafford Farms, Inc.

Paid Medical Claims

	Paid claims	Exposures	Average claims per employee
Period A 10/1/85 10/1/86	$2,287,783	28,973	$ 78.96
Period B 10/1/86 10/1/87	2,925,788	27,340	107.01
Period A	78.96×1.131*=89.30		
Period B	107.01×1.202*=128.63		

$$\frac{B-A}{A} = \frac{123.84 - 89.30}{89.30} = +44.04\%$$

*Trend.

Table 5-8. Stafford Farms, Inc.

Noninstitutional Services from 1986 through June 1, 1988—Average Charges for Services

Service type	Nonpreferred			Preferred		
	1986	1987	1988	1986	1987	1988
Medical	$ 38.95	$ 43.49	$ 44.48	$ 30.24	$ 35.65	$ 35.02
Surgery	278.81	316.18	300.95	142.02	177.96	210.14
Psychiatric	67.15	72.15	75.72	82.93	77.45	84.63
X ray and lab	35.32	41.00	46.97	18.78	19.44	20.67
Anesthesia	376.42	406.52	439.32	257.94	310.73	296.06
Radiology	50.00	63.25	47.48	42.99	47.02	39.55
Injections	13.86	15.39	33.34	13.93	16.44	19.01
Assistant surgeon	538.30	309.17	465.17	223.18	225.65	234.86
Other services	109.62	61.31	83.60	12.40	15.92	41.28
Total	$ 65.57	$ 63.60	$ 68.38	$ 34.72	$ 40.02	$ 45.97
Percentage change		−3	+7		+15	+15

Table 5-9 indicates that between 1986 and 1987 there was a 19 percent increase in noninstitutional or nonhospital services. The use of these services is largely determined by patient demand and physician practice patterns. The total number of medical services delivered jumped from 16 services per insured in 1986 to 20 in 1987. This is three times the expected level of services per insured. The carrier had no explanation

Table 5-9. Stafford Farms, Inc.

Number of Services Used

	1986	1987	1988
Medical	15,003	17,600	18,830
Surgical	2,283	2,366	2,438
Psychiatric	4,639	5,722	6,480
X ray and lab	7,558	11,051	11,530
Anesthesia	258	241	245
Radiology	1,045	1,060	1,046
Injections	1,444	1,668	1,692
Assistant surgeon	70	89	65
Other services	6,096	5,802	2,654
Total	38,396	45,598	44,981
Percentage change	N/A	+19%	−1%
Percentage number of insureds	2,421	2,287	2,287
Services per insured (average)	16	20	20

for this dramatic increase other than to blame employees for overusing the plan and to cite the 1 percent decline in usage.

Stafford realized that it had little control over these costs since the PPO consisted of over 95 percent of the physicians in the area (all the physicians belonging to the local IPA). When the IPA was presented with the usage and fees figures, the response was that there was little that could be done since the employees asked for the services and the doctors often had to provide more extended visits to guard against potential malpractice claims.

Besides the spiraling outpatient costs, hospital costs were also on the rise. Table 5-10 illustrates that between 1984 and 1986, the number of admissions dropped slightly and the number of days dropped significantly. However, by 1988 hospital usage was back to 1984 levels. This was of great concern to Stafford Farms' insurance committee because standard medical practice at the time was to move less severely ill pa-

Table 5-10. Stafford Farms, Inc.

Inpatient Hospital Use Report

Hospital use per 1000 insured	1984	1985	1986	1987	1988
Number of admissions	79	91	72	80	80
Number of days	426	466	301	383	430
Average stay (days)	5.4	5.1	4.2	4.8	5.4

Table 5-11. Stafford Farms, Inc.
Total Costs

Year ending 9/30	1984	1985	1986	1987	1988
Medical benefits (× 100)	$1611	$2079	$2566	$3162	$3602
Change over previous year	—	29%	23%	23%	14%
General fund increase	10.9%	4.6%	7.3%	10.1%	5.4%
Consumer Price Index (CPI)	4.3%	3.6%	2.0%	4.4%	4.0%

tients to outpatient settings, thereby reducing the number and duration of hospital stays. The number of admissions should have been declining while outpatient care was increasing.

Finally, Stafford Farms compared total medical benefits costs for the last 5 years with operating budget increases and the consumer price index (CPI). This information is contained in Table 5-11.

The increase in benefits cost was consistently greater than the increases in the operating fund. In order to control costs, the Stafford's committee realized that such items as the $100 deductible, the $5 copays for office visits, the stop-loss provision of $2500, and the way in which the carrier was coordinating benefits would need to be changed in order to control usage. In addition, because of the high psychiatric, chiropractic, and inpatient costs, covered services would have to be redesigned in such a manner as to continue to provide the catastrophic coverage desired by employees while holding the line on premium costs.

Demanding and Implementing Change

It was apparent that some immediate changes had to be instituted to bring spiraling costs under control. In 1988, Stafford Farms demanded and received changes in plan design which would control the excessive use of nonhospital services. However, it soon became clear that the plan design changes did little more than hold the line on costs. Further, spiraling premium costs were making the carrier question whether it even wanted to remain as the insurer for Stafford. A radical redesign of the medical benefits plan was needed. Therefore, it was going to be important for Stafford's insurance committee, working with carriers and consultants, to radically redesign the plan in order to control health care costs.

Consultants' Advice. The consultants suggested several changes in plan design. But, as had already been realized, making changes in the amount of patient copays and modifications to the stop-loss provisions would be insufficient to remedy the growing problem. These changes would help control usage by employees but not address the shift toward higher coding of office visits by providers. Analysis of the data indicated that cost-containment strategies with the PPO network and tighter case management would also have to be put into place. Much of this would have to be done by the carrier.

Carrier's Case Management. Of immediate concern to the committee was the way in which claims were being processed by the carrier. It appeared that claims processors were serving as conduits, merely forwarding Stafford's premium dollars directly to the providers with little or no case management. The carrier was relying solely on Stafford employees for information regarding eligibility. There were no preexisting condition clauses and no safeguards to ensure that total (aggregate) claims running more than $10,000 to $15,000 were being managed. It was not until individual medical expenses exceeded $50,000 for a specific diagnosis that the carrier began to examine individual claims.

It also became clear that the carrier was doing little if anything to control or question the fees charged by providers. Claims processors were using the standard of usual and customary charges as the primary control of doctors' fees. There was no control over the number of office visits and ancillary treatments. Simply, there were no safeguards to manage patient utilization and service charges other than preadmission authorization.

This information on how the claims were being processed in conjunction with the data obtained on the plans performance was shared with the carrier and the providers. While the carrier and the providers had some suggestions for plan design changes, their immediate reaction was that the primary problem was Stafford's employees' overuse of the plan. The providers believed that the carrier was also at fault for not providing them with more information to use in conducting internal audits. They were unwilling to accept any culpability in the matter, referring to all plan design changes as the employer's responsibility.

Designing a New Plan. What developed was a finger-pointing situation in which no one group was willing to assume its share of blame for the problem. The carrier and the providers blamed the employees, the providers blamed the employees and the carrier, the carrier blamed the employees and the providers, and employees were beginning to feel threatened.

At this point, the insurance committee faced new challenges and obligations. Initially, the committee wished to resolve the problem with the existing carrier and providers. The unwillingness of the carrier and providers to develop a joint solution to the problem, however, provided the insurance committee with additional insight into what it needed to accomplish. Armed with this information, it began to work toward devising options for a new plan design.

As insurance committees begin to look at the present and possible future designs of their organizations, medical benefits program, they should request the documents described in the following focus guide. Some committees will not need every report, while others may have need for additional reports designed specifically for a particular organization.

Focus Guide

Research Documents

Any employer wishing to conduct an analysis of plan design costs should secure from the current carrier the following documentation:

- Summary of benefits.
- Monthly claims (loss ratio) report.
- A list of plan design changes that have been instituted for the previous 3 years and how they compare with the design of the current plan.
- Total of premium, detailed by individual, spouse, and children.
- Total premium cost for the employer and total premium cost for the employee for the current year to date, as well as for the projected year and the previous 3 years.
- A total claims summary by CPT4 and by line of coverage including increases or decreases for the previous 3 years.
- Hospital utilization summary for the previous 3 years by admitted diagnosis, length of stay, inpatient, outpatient, and ambulatory figures.
- A summary of utilization for the previous 3 years by preferred and nonpreferred provider or by exclusive preferred and nonpreferred if these are options within the plan.
- A breakdown of the number and cost of office visits and their increase or decrease for the previous 3 years.
- A diagnostic-related group (DRG) report. This report may appear under any of several titles. It shows inpatient and outpatient utiliza-

tion at hospitals including average length of stay by hospital, average length of stay by a major diagnostic category, average hospital charges by major diagnostic categories, and average length of stay by patient as prescribed by physicians.

- Specific costs for inpatient and outpatient treatment of mental nervous disorder for the previous 3 years broken down by dependent versus employee use.

The premium and total claims loss ratio reports should be received by an employer on a monthly basis. Any reports dealing with summary of benefits or summaries over a 3-year period should be provided on a quarterly or semiannual basis for the current year, with previous years information on an annual basis. If an employer has not been receiving these reports and conducting an analysis of them on a routine basis, it will be necessary to gather them together, and then to place future reviews on a scheduled basis.

6
Initiating Changes in Your Health Care Plan

How to Initiate Change

Once all the data have been sufficiently reviewed, it becomes possible to make changes to ensure that the plan will be more cost-efficient. However, before changes are initiated, a thorough analysis of your utilization patterns over the previous 3 years, as described in Chapter 5, should be conducted, along with an employee survey (see Appendix B). Without this analysis and data, it will be impossible to redesign the plan to contain costs while still meeting the needs of employees. If the plan design analysis yields results similar to those presented in Chapter 5, as many analyses do, design changes will likely focus on shifting greater cost for the program onto the employee, shifting responsibility for accurate case management onto the carrier, and limiting the number of preferred providers offered through the plan, while meeting specific needs of employees as shown in the survey. Penalties for the carrier's failure carrier to comply should be built into the plan design.

Plan Redesign Initiated by Committee Consensus

Insurance committee participation and consensus are essential when a company is considering proposed plan design changes. While no employee likes to see reduced benefits, employees should be in a position to understand and agree that increased costs for reduced benefits are harmful and unacceptable. When committee members are given hard data that indicate the need for change, they will probably be supportive if the proposed cost shifting does not also mean increased premiums for reduced benefits and if the redesign mirrors employees' needs as reflected in the survey. At the very least, employees should come to understand the complexity of medical benefits costs and be better equipped to make educated decisions regarding the extent and costs of the coverage they need. These costs should be weighed against dollars available for employee pay increases, and employees can make decisions about whether to take increases in salary or in benefits.

The Role of Outside Consultants during the Redesign Phase

During the redesign process, outside, independent consultants can be extremely useful. They can review the data with the committee and discuss alternatives to the current plan design. Figure 6-1 contains an agenda used by an insurance committee that was struggling with plan design. As a result of this meeting, which included an outside consultant, the company's broker, and representatives from the current carrier, radical changes in the current plan were proposed by the committee.

The Need for Carrier Cost Management

The committee also discussed the need for stronger case management on the part of the carrier. The committee agreed that if the current carrier could not provide the level of case management sought, the organization should go to bid for a new carrier or a case-management firm. If a case-management firm was retained, the cost for such services was to come from the carrier's retention fees. Obviously, not all committees will come to these same decisions. The demographics, needs, and utilization of different organizations differ. If the actual medical claims are running approximately 75 percent of the premium (a low loss ratio), and if the employees are generally satisfied with the plan, then no changes should be made. The old maxim "If it isn't broken, don't fix it" applies.

Insurance Meeting
Agenda

Purposes of the Insurance Committee Meeting

1. To review history (design, coverages, cost, utilization) of current insurance plans
2. To review results of insurance survey
3. To understand the budget in regard to insurance
4. To provide overview of national insurance norms and trends
5. To make proposed plan design decisions

Tuesday Morning

1. Welcome and introductions
   BARBARA KLANTZ, *Human Resources Division*

   - Review purposes
   - Review agenda

2. Overview of history of insurance plans
   DAVE WAGNER, *Carrier Representative*

   a. History of medical and dental plan
      - Design
      - Coverages
      - Cost
      - Utilization
   b. Company role in medical-dental plan
   c. Long-term disability (LTD) plan

3. Budget implications
   THERESA BLUM, *Accounting*

   a. Historical costs
   b. Increases: 1987 and 1988
   c. Budgetary limitations

Tuesday Afternoon

4. Results of insurance survey
   BILL BRAXTON, *Consultant*

   a. Overall
   b. By group
   c. Comments

Figure 6-1. Insurance meeting agenda.

5. National trends and norms in insurance
   BILL BRAXTON

6. Objectives for insurance plan design
   BILL BRAXTON

7. Plan design issues
   BILL BRAXTON

   a. Preexisting conditions
   b. Discretionary services
   c. Maintenance services
   d. Internal equities
   e. Preferred risk pool
   f. High technology
   g. Ethics

Wednesday

8. Plan design suggestions
9. Next steps

Figure 6-1. (*Continued*)

Committee Involvement in Rebidding

However, even if there is no need to rebid or redesign the plan, it is essential to keep the insurance committee involved on a regular basis in reviewing reports and monitoring employee needs. The committee member's role as a communicator with other staff members about the importance of prudent use of medical care should not be minimized. Open channels of communication between management and staff are essential for maintenance of positive relations and smooth operating principles.

Rebidding as a Matter of Course

Even when a particular medical benefits plan is working efficiently, some consultants recommend that companies routinely rebid their programs every 3 to 4 years in order to ensure that they are getting good value for their money. This recommended rebidding applies to fully insured programs and self-insured programs using administrative services only (ASO), or third-party administrators (TPAs). While going to bid can assist an employer in finding out whether the company is receiving good value for its dollar, the process can also cost thousands of dollars. It should be remembered that the advice to rebid often comes from consultants who stand to gain financially from the rebidding process.

Ledeke Enterprises: Rebidding a Master Contract

Ledeke Enterprises is a family-owned business with several auto repair franchises throughout the Southeast. The Ledeke family prides itself on its ability to "take care of our own," and the company president, Al Ledeke, is in full agreement with the family's philosophy. Ledeke has traditionally offered reasonable wages and a strong package of employee benefits to his 3600 workers.

Late last year the manager of the organization's Tampa muffler shop suffered a cerebral hemorrhage. Rehabilitation costs were astronomical. The plan covered catastrophic illnesses, but the Ledekes discovered that the employee's family had paid nearly $4000 in out-of-pocket expenses prior to reaching the stop-loss. Al Ledeke personally authorized reimbursement to the family out of company funds. Following this incident, Ledeke retained the services of an insurance consultant to evaluate the company's medical benefits program.

The consultant reviewed the master contract and advised that the current program was sufficient for employees' needs—including provisions for catastrophic illness such as the manager's hemorrhage. The Ledekes' choice to supplement medical services was made out of loyalty to their employees, and did not reflect a deficit in the insurance program. Despite the positive evaluation, the consultant suggested rebidding the insurance contract "just to see what would shake loose." He explained that rebidding would enable Ledeke to be sure that it was getting the best possible return on the company's investment dollar.

Reluctantly, Al Ledeke agreed to the rebidding. After 6 months of examining options, approving requests for bid, and reviewing proposals, Ledeke Enterprises signed a new contract, incorporating minor plan design changes, with the same carrier as it had used for the previous 6 years. The total cost for this process was in excess of $7500.

The Dangers of Routine Rebidding

Despite consultants' frequent advice to the contrary, rebidding is not an activity to be initiated without first thoroughly considering the associated costs. An organization with approximately 3200 employees that is rebidding a single medical plan should budget between $4000 and $7000 to cover the costs associated with preparing the request for proposals and analysis of bids, if an outside consultant is used. The more complex the plan or options, and the larger the organization, the higher the cost of rebidding. Smaller employers, who cannot get experience-rated plans, will not have to budget these funds because the cost of the rebidding will be built into the broker's commission. The smaller employers should pay close attention to their broker's commission and retention fees to determine the actual cost of rebidding.

Alternatives to Rebidding

Other methods besides rebidding can help employers to determine whether they are receiving good value for their medical benefits dollars. For example, comparable organizations and plans within the same geographic area can be reviewed by a consultant. The cost of this service is far less than rebidding.

Determining whether Rebidding Is Appropriate

An organization experiencing any of the following should consider rebidding the master contract as one available option.

- The monthly claims experience is resulting in an extremely high loss ratio of 90 percent (or more) of the total premium on an annualized basis.
- The premiums are rising above the national trend.
- The organization is considering a move from a fully self-insured plan with internal administration to a self-insured plan with a TPA.
- The organization is moving from a fully insured plan to a partially self-insured plan.
- Federal and state regulations require changes in plan design.
- There is a high level of employee and management dissatisfaction with the present carrier.

If an organization is faced with any of the conditions described above, changes should be made. What should be avoided is making major changes quickly and inefficiently. If possible, either the plan design or the carrier should be changed, but not both at the same time. As many organizations have discovered, this is not always possible.

If it appears that both plan design and carrier must be changed, employees may be adversely affected unless employee education regarding forthcoming changes is clear and timely. Even with this preparatory education, staff members involved in managing the benefits program will spend a great amount of time during the first 6 months of the plan clarifying misconceptions and working directly with employee concerns.

Rebidding and the Current Carrier

Prior to making the decision to change plan design through rebidding, an employer should forward a list of the plan design changes to the current carrier. The carrier should be given the opportunity to incorporate the plan design changes, including case management and plan administration changes, into the existing policy. If the carrier indicates that such changes are possible, you should determine whether the proposed redesign does in fact meet the company's needs and will help curb costs incurred by the organization. Also determine what risk the carrier is willing to take to ensure that implemented changes work.

Because plan design changes are based on utilization review data, and are aimed at correcting the problems of misuse and overuse, the carrier should be willing to work with the employer to stabilize or lower premiums. However, if the carrier seems unwilling or unable to control costs through case-management procedures, the employer should go to bid rather than wasting time on fruitless negotiation.

Paulist Hills Water Conservation District: Seeking Carrier Cooperation in Controlling Costs

The Paulist Hills Water Conservation District was in the process of redesigning its medical benefits plan in an effort to cut back on costs. Working with a consultant, the governing board of the district developed a list of plan design changes the members wished to institute. A list of these changes (Figure 6-2) was forwarded to the existing carrier with a cover letter detailing the district's reasons for seeking the changes.

The carrier responded to this request by projecting a 9.2 percent increase in premium costs over the current design. The carrier also reserved the right to adjust the increase based on a review of use during the months prior to renewal. While this, combined with a 9.2 percent increase, does not at first seem unreasonable, the resulting

---

Phase 2 Insurance Study

Recommendations for phase 2 of the insurance study are as follows.

1. *Goals.* Approve the goals adopted by the insurance committee.

2. *FSA.* Establish an FSA that allows individual staff members to pay pretax dollars for otherwise uncovered medical, dental, vision, or child care premiums, or for additional medical or life insurance premiums.

3. *PPO changes.* Change the PPO from a $15 copay to a $100 deductible; thereafter the insurance company picks up 80 percent of all costs to the current stop-loss amount, of $5000.

   The maximum mental health benefit for PPO outpatient care will be 50 percent of charges up to $1250 per year. This will not count toward stop loss.

   The maximum chiropractor benefit will be 50 percent of charges up to $500 per year. This will not count toward stop loss.

4. *Indemnity plan changes.* Change the indemnity plan from the current $100 deductible to a $250 deductible with the insurance company picking up 70 percent of all costs thereafter up to a $7500 stop loss. Nonhospital indemnity plan service provided by medical doctors will be reimbursed at 70 percent of costs.

   Maximum mental health benefits for outpatient care will remain at 50 percent of charges up to a maximum of $1250 per year and will continue not to count toward stop loss.

   Maximum chiropractic benefits will be at 50 percent of charges to a maximum of $500 per year and will continue to not count toward stop loss.

   Medical doctor, nonhospital services will be reimbursed at 70 percent of charges. These charges *will* count toward stop loss.

5. *Plan administration costs.*

   Request the insurance carrier to reduce the number of PPOs and refine the criteria for selecting PPO physicians, hospitals, and other service providers. This will tighten utilization management, costs, and claims administration.

   Change the coordination-of-benefits provision to a "carve-out" provision.

Figure 6-2. Proposed recommendations for final report.

Request that the medical insurance carrier tighten management and administration of the benefit plan to include case management for any claim with cumulative charges in excess of $10,000 per year.

Require the insurance carrier to conduct precertification and concurrent review for all PPO and non-PPO hospital admissions.

Require preauthorization review for all outpatient surgeries or any other treatments or procedures which cost in excess of a dollar limit (e.g., $500) determined by the employer and the carrier to be appropriate.

Require the carrier to review all hospital admissions and the results of preadmission concurrent reviews with the employer on a monthly basis for the fiscal year.

Limit transplants in both plans to procedures that are routinely accepted in medical practice, e.g., kidney transplants, bone marrow transplants. Require the carrier to contract with specific providers for all provided transplant services using a "centers-for-excellence" approach.

Exclude peripheral practitioners' charges from the plan, e.g., rolfers, naturopaths, herbalists.

Request the carrier to provide quarterly cost and utilization reports in addition to the rolling charges monthly report.

Require the carrier to provide booklets describing the new summary plan descriptions (booklets) for all staff by January 1.

6. *Full flexible benefits.* Study full flexible benefits and the impact of adding additional options such as an HMO. This study should be completed by the first quarter of 1989 so that recommendations can be implemented by January 1.

7. *Benefits manager.* Hire a full-time professional technical person to coordinate benefits administration and to provide information and education to employees.

Figure 6-2. (*Continued*)

increase in potential costs to employees by 35 percent does seem unreasonable. The district and the insurance committee realized this and asked the carrier to assume some risk by holding at a 0 percent increase (Figure 6-3).

The carrier's rationale for the increase was the need to offset

Prerenewal Statement

. The Paulist Hills Water Conservation District requested that
The Insurance Source of the West (ISW) provide a prerenewal
commitment for January 1. Following is a summary of the information we can provide to date regarding our renewal as-
sumptions.

Current renewal estimate:

Medical: 25.8%

Dental: Current rate base (CRB)

Overall: 21.1%

As an alternative to a renewal commitment, we can provide a
renewal commitment to the above estimates with the assumption that medical claims do not exceed $831,000 for the 3
months from August through October of the previous year combined and that dental claims do not exceed $120,000 during the
same period. If claims exceed these limits, or if they are significantly lower, ISW will have the right to revise the renewal.

Additionally, Paulist Hills Water Conservation District and its
consultants requested that we review the following renewal
plan design and administrative modifications for January 1 and
the resulting savings.

Figure 6-3. Response from carrier for renewal bid.

trend and to build up reserves because of the high loss ratio the
plan had incurred over the previous 3 years. The board had felt all
along that the high loss ratio was caused by changes initiated by the
carrier over the previous 3 years and that, therefore, the carrier
should share in the responsibility for the problem. One way in

	Plan design change	Credit
1. PPO	$100 deductible 80/20 on the next $5000.	−5.2%
Non-PPO	$250 deductible	
	Hospital charges at 80/20% on the next $7500. All other non-PPO charges are at 70%.	
2. Chiropractic limitation set at 50% to a maximum of $500 per year		−2.3
3. Precertification and concurrent review for both PPO and non-PPO		−3.0
4. Carve-out in place of standard coordination of benefits (COB)		−0.5
5. Mental and nervous limitations		
$1000 limit		−1.0
$1250 limit		0.5
6. * Total credit for modifications		−12.0
* Estimated renewal (medical and dental) of current plan from page 1		+21.1
* Combined medical and dental rate increase adjusted for plan changes		+09.2

The plan design and administrative modifications do not include the proposed modifications listed below, which may provide additional savings. These modifications were still being evaluated at the time of producing this report.

* Provider fee freeze and/or PPO provider negotiations
* Potential hospitalization discounts that may be negotiated before January.

Figure 6-3. (*Continued*)

which the carrier could do this would be to build the reserves more slowly than it had indicated it wished, and another way was to institute tighter case management and plan administration.

After several months of negotiations, it became clear that even with radical plan design changes, the carrier would still request an increase. In fact, during the final weeks of negotiation the carrier demanded a 20 percent increase due to continued high loss ratios. During the same period, the carrier indicated that it had failed to case-manage several large claims, as the district had requested it to do. As a result, Paulist Hills Water Conservation District went to bid for a new carrier and a new plan design.

Defining the Goals of a Benefits Program

As an organization begins to plan for change, members of the insurance committee must determine that the goals of the benefits program reflect what the proposed plan design changes are attempting to do. Ideally, these goals should have been adopted by the committee early in its work. Figure 6-4 shows one example of a set of goals. These goals will assist in softening the effect of the data on employees and employee groups. Employer-provided medical benefit plans have become highly emotional issues. Using these goals, the data that have been gathered from the utilization review and survey, along with the proposed plan design changes, allow the employer to prepare for the change on the basis of facts rather than emotion. The data also enable the committee to work more efficiently with the consultant as it assists in preparing the request for proposal.

---

1. To determine the best coverage possible for all employees within the parameters of the money available for insurance

2. To structure the medical and dental plans so that increases in premiums for the company and the company's employees do not exceed the CPI

3. To examine all present insurance benefits available to employees, so as to put together a sound, cost-effective package of benefits

4. To keep employees informed about the insurance committee's work, including (a) the reasons for making adjustments to insurance offerings and (b) what to expect in the insurance field

5. To recommend an insurance package for implementation which meets the expressed needs of staff within the parameters available for insurance

6. To make employees more sensitive to the cost of medical services so that they will become better consumers of these services

---

Figure 6-4. Goals of the benefits program.

Preparing the Bid

Unless the organization is extremely large, with full-time attorneys and actuaries, and with highly trained benefits specialists, an outside consulting firm should be employed to prepare the bid. The bid should include:

- The overall goals of the benefits plan
- Requests for all special reports to be delivered to the company and its insurance committee on a scheduled basis
- The type of case management desired
- The type of funding requested in the plan, such as maximum termination liability (MTL)
- A description of the existing plan design and funding
- A description of the proposed plan design
- Demographics on all plan participants, including a definition of all eligible participants
- Available statistics on the utilization and the cost of the benefits provided
- A request for a "no-loss, no-gain" provision which states that the new carrier is responsible for taking on all currently covered plan participants and cannot subject these participants to eligibility requirements nor reduce their benefits beyond the level of those proposed in the plan

Establishing a Realistic Time Frame

It should take up to 4 weeks for a consultant to prepare the specifications of the bid and to review them with the insurance committee. The specifications should be carefully reviewed by members of the insurance committee prior to distribution by the consultant. If the plan design provisions and bid specifications are not in keeping with the organization's proposed changes, the bidding process will obviously not yield the expected results.

Another 4 to 6 weeks should be allocated for the various carriers to respond. Once the deadline for receiving the proposal has been met, the consultant should prepare a summary chart for each proposal and each aspect of the plan design for review by the committee. Based on this comparison, which should also include a comparison of premium

rates, it should be possible to select the individual carriers the committee wishes to interview. Figure 6-5 includes an outline form that can be
used to compare various insurance carriers.

Interviewing Potential Carriers

At least 2 hours should be set aside for each carrier interview. It is recommended that the entire insurance committee or overseeing body of
the insurance committee be present during the interviews. The consultant who prepares the bid specifications should also be present. A specific set of questions should be prepared for the interview and used with
all finalists. A sample set of questions is shown in Figure 6-6. These
questions are intended to provide a general outline from which to work.
Specific questions pertaining to a particular organization should be
written by members of the insurance committee. In addition, the consultants should provide separate questions dealing with technical funding provisions of the policy.

How the Carrier Manages Care and
Controls Costs

Of particular concern to company representatives who interview insurance carriers should be the manner in which the carriers deal with managing care and cost containment. Carriers who claim to have a large
number of preferred providers available who accept lower fees for eligible participants should be closely queried about how they are able to
effectively manage such a large and diverse network of providers and
how they guard against code creep and unbundling.

The Size of PPO Networks Can
Adversely Affect Costs

Effective control of the costs of individual doctors who are part of a
large PPO network is difficult. For example, one employer used a PPO
network which included the physicians in the area who belonged to the
IPA. The 450 doctors in the plan included 90 to 95 percent of the physicians in the area. When the loss ratio for the plan began to exceed 100
percent and the doctors' fees rose 15 percent, it became clear to the
employer that one way to control costs was to use a smaller network of
doctors.

Organizations working through the rebidding process should not hes-

1. Preliminary screening criteria

   a. Summary of benefits
      (1) Deductibles
      (2) Coinsurance
      (3) Lifetime maximum
      (4) Limitations
      (5) Cost-management programs

   b. Benefits cost and design compatibility
      (1) Premium costs
         - Paid premium
         - Paid claims
         - IBNR reserve
         - Pooling charge
         - Total incurred
         - Retention
           Taxes
           Commission
           All other
         - Total retention
         - Percentage of premium
         - Dividend or surplus
         - Assumptions
           Incurred loss ratio
           Pooling
           Interest credit
           Paid claims
      (2) Benefits comparability to bid specifications

   c. Historical development
      (1) Organizational structure
         - Type: ownership or board
         - Management or staff experiences
         - Administrative integration
         - Provider references
      (2) Operating philosophy
         - Clarity and consistency
         - Compatibility with internal goals
      (3) Provider network
         - Geographic territory
         - Adequacy of services
         - How selected

Figure 6-5. Summary analysis of carrier finalists.

(4) Commitment
- Local presence, size, and market posture
- Financial investment
- Risk assumption flexibility

2. Secondary screening criteria
   a Management capabilities
      (1) Provider selection criteria
      (2) Provider reimbursement
         - For indemnity
         - For PPO or EPO
      (3) Employee satisfaction systems
         - Patient information; patient advocacy
         - Employee education
         - Appeal complaint process
      (4) Management information systems
         - Unit cost variations
         - Reports available
         - Practice pattern variations
         - Inpatient hospital use
           Preadmission review
           Concurrent review
           Case management
           Special reviews
         - Managed care components
      (5) Others specific to your bid (e.g., FSAs)

Figure 6.5. (*Continued*)

itate to convey to insurance carriers their desire to limit the size of the provider network. In some instances carriers will be willing to convert their current HMO network of doctors into a PPO network for a specific plan and to provide indemnity access to these doctors. Insurance committees should be creative and not be afraid to ask in an interview what special arrangements the carrier can make. Just as the plan design changes were made to specifically target areas of overuse, the carrier's plan-management needs must also be in line. This may require creation of a plan tailored to your specific needs. Carriers should be willing to meet the specific needs of their clients. However, due to differing insurance regulations among the states with regard to filed rates, funding, and operations, a carrier may not be able to address specific needs. If a carrier is unable to meet your needs, e.g., reducing the number of doctors in its network, and it is the committee's feeling that a smaller

1. How large an organization are you? Can you deliver needed services within the area? How are out-of-state services handled?

2. Explain your hospital precertification procedures. Why are employee patients required to precertify?

3. How do you control the frequency of utilization? How do you control code creep and unbundling of charges by providers?

4. How is case management handled?
   - Do you use on-site case review?
   - Do your case managers interface with claims processing records?
   - How do you determine which cases are managed?
     By admitting diagnosis
     By accumulated cost
     By the individual
     Other (specify)

5. How do you handle claims submitted for medical services that were provided out of state? (Note that this question has major significance for organizations that employ traveling salespeople or representatives. Many of the claims submitted by these employees may come from out of state.)

6. What is the experience of your staff? Will this account have "dedicated" claims personnel, people working only on this account? If this plan design has unique features, how do you intend to train your staff to enforce them? How will mistakes be handled?

7. How can you limit rate increases by the following providers?
   - Physicians
   - Hospitals
   - Other service providers

8. What reports are available on a monthly, quarterly, and annual basis? What clients may we call to review the types of reports provided to them?

9. How flexible are you about redesigning your plan to correct future utilization or cost problems as well as service problems?

10. What kind of employee communication information is available to the employer? Is there a cost associated with this information?

11. What kind of consumer education and assistance do you provide? Do you have an 800 number which employees can call for answers to questions?

Figure 6-6. Carrier finalist interview questions.

12. How many flexible spending accounts (FSAs) do you currently administer?

13. How frequently do you pay out of the FSA accounts to employees? How frequently do you provide a summary of account to employees?

14. How do you explain your retention fees and your termination liability?

Cautions

- Look for direct, honest answers that address your problems.
- Be cautious about patronizing self-serving statements.
- Be careful about showmanship and "media" techniques. Look at the content of the answers and what makes sense for the organization and employees.

Additional Questions about HMOs

1. What HMO benefit plans are available to our company? What are the options that exist within each of the HMO plans you offer? Can you provide information on current enrollment figures for each plan? Can you give us a list of other employers in the area using these plans?

2. What methods does your company use to make available to an employer information on the positive or negative impact of selecting the indemnity plan? The HMO option?

3. What methods does your company routinely employ to measure:

- Employee satisfaction with the HMO?
- Quality of care provided by the HMO?
- Access to the HMO?

4. How many of your HMO doctors are board-certified? How are physicians reimbursed? Are there incentives to induce them to skimp on care?

5. Can our employees choose the HMO doctors they prefer? How long does it take to get an appointment? How difficult is it to consult with a specialist?

6. What documentation can you provide about the quality of the hospital with which your HMO is affiliated?

Figure 6.6. (*Continued*)

number of doctors or HMO is necessary in order to control costs, then you should look for a different carrier.

The Carrier's Cost-Management Practices

Another issue which should receive close scrutiny when you are interviewing potential carriers is the types of cost-management practices that are available. The checklist in Figure 6-7 includes many items that should be considered. Questions specifically relating to an employer's program should be added when appropriate.

Other Cost-Management Practices.   Other cost-management practices include well-baby programs for expectant mothers, preferred pharmacy options, and on-site case management of all hospital admissions. A special case is use of "centers for excellence"; the carrier contracts with specific institutions for such procedures as organ transplants and open-heart surgery because these institutions have the best track records for effective and efficient service. It is less expensive to treat plan participants at such centers, even if airfare must be paid, than it is to have them treated at local institutions which do not have the experienced staff or facilities to perform such complicated procedures.

- Audits of hospital and doctor bills
- Concurrent review and discharge planning
- Home health care benefits
- Hospice benefits
- Hospital length-of-stay assignments
- Incentives for outpatient surgery
- Incentives for outpatient diagnostic and preadmission tests
- Individual case management
- Weekend admission limitations
- Long-term custodial care
- Precertification and preadmission review programs
- Second opinions prior to surgery
- Wellness benefits

Figure 6-7. Potential carrier considerations.

In this era of advancing medical technology and costs, it is prudent to be leery of any carrier who is able to deliver only precertification and preadmission review and second-surgical-opinion programs. The more "hands-on" case management that is provided, such as prenatal workups and visits to hospitalized staff members by registered nurses, the better the program will be for covered employees. If the carrier is unable to provide a high level of case management and plan administration, it should be willing to reduce the premium so that an outside case-management service can be retained. The carrier should be familiar with several such organizations and may wish to contract directly for these services, or may leave the contracting for services up to the employer.

The Role and Purpose of Flexible Spending Accounts

If an organization is adding FSAs to the benefits plan, the carrier should be able to explain clearly how it intends to administer the accounts, if administration is included in the bid. While FSAs offer tax savings for employees and employers, they can cause problems if a lag develops between the time employees deposit funds into their accounts and the time plan administrators write checks for child-care or medical expense accounts.

New Rules in 1990

In addition, as of January 1990 employers must bear some of the risk incumbent in FSAs. They must treat health care expenses under FSAs like life insurance. That is, if an employee elects to place $100 a month into a health expense account and incurs $1200 of expenses during the first calendar month, the complete $1200 must be reimbursed even though only $100 is in the account. This will cause more employers to rethink the feasibility of FSAs. However, even if the employer drops this feature, dependent care and premium accounts can be retained as before.

The Remnants of the Tax Reform Act

Although the Tax Reform Act—Section 89 of the Internal Revenue Code (IRC)—has been repealed, it is prudent for an employer to use the tests in Section 89 as guidelines for their benefits plans. These tests also apply to any company which must follow Employee Retirement Insurance Act (ERISA) guidelines. Further, the issue of highly compensated employees will likely reappear in the near future. The relevant tests are listed below.

Test 1.   The plan must be in writing. Eligibility and benefits must be clearly stated.

Test 2.   Employees must have legally enforceable rights under the plan.

Test 3.   Employees must be notified in writing of the summary plan description.

Test 4.   The plan must be for the sole benefit of the employees.

Test 5.   The plan must be established and maintained by the employer on an indefinite basis.

As an organization moves toward selecting a new carrier, the proposed plan design should be examined in light of these five tests, which are actually more complicated than they might first appear. The carrier and the consultants should, however, be in a position to assist clients with presenting the information to employees in clear language, meeting these tests.

Final Interviews

Last-Minute Negotiations by Senior Insurance Committee Members

If the committee is still concerned about specific aspects of competing plans after the interviews, it is suggested that the consultant and/or employer call each finalist to review the considerations and to request adjustments. Some consultants, however, especially those working with large national consulting firms, are uncomfortable with this procedure, as it may be difficult to keep track of decisions and promises made under such circumstances. It may be more efficient to have a senior representative of the insurance committee conduct this last round of negotiations. The final outcomes of the telephone negotiations should be followed up in writing and should meet the general specifications of the bid.

Carrier Participation

Carriers should, ideally, be willing to conduct last-minute negotiations, recognizing that a company engaged in an in-depth benefits analysis is signaling its assurance that it is truly interested in cutting costs and becoming partners in providing effective coverage. In addition, carriers should be aware that the committee and the employees it represents have high expectations with regard to plan administration, cost containment, and the manner in which the provider network operates. However, it appears that some insurance companies regard intense scrutiny to be an invasion of their field of expertise. They prefer to design, administer, and alter insurance programs internally rather than in partnership with clients. If you are interested in working closely with your carrier, it is in your best interest to find a carrier willing to commit the time and effort necessary.

Reference Checks

The committee should be willing to take the time to check references. It should ask a potential carrier for a list of current clients, and then should ask the clients about the carrier's case-management practices, sensitivity to employee needs, and general organization and functioning. Even though a carrier may have developed a very attractive proposal, it may be falling short in servicing existing plans. If so, the company should reconsider carefully before signing a contract.

Given all of the above information—the responses to the questions, the review of the carrier's case-management and cost-containment practices, and any information arising as a result of last-minute negotiations—the committee should be able to make a decision about its recommended carrier. It is essential that top management be supportive of the final outcome of this decision. As the committee makes the final deliberation, the exact premium costs should not be the most important consideration, if in fact the costs are approximately what the company is looking for. It is extremely difficult for a carrier to accurately predict the actual cost of a plan design for a company for which the carrier has not previously provided coverage, and the task becomes even more difficult if there have been radical plan design changes. If the projected costs are close to what you are looking for, it is possible to negotiate the actual rates you wish, especially if the carrier realizes you are willing to work cooperatively to control costs. Of greater concern to committee members should be the management and philosophy of the carrier, the provider reimbursement procedures, the selection method for the doctors, the geographic coverage and access for employees, the management practices in relationship to the preferred provider network, and the overall services which the carrier appears to be willing to provide (including frequency of comunication with the employer and the availability of reports to help the employer work toward meeting the objectives of the plan).

Major Changes Should Be Carefully Orchestrated

If the committee has decided to rebid and to make radical plan design changes, the changes should be made as carefully and expediently as possible. Phasing plan design changes in gradually over a 3-year period has the potential of causing greater upheaval among employees than does making one drastic plan redesign, such as changing the carrier and significantly shifting costs. Once employees recognize that their out-of-pocket costs for premium contributions and/or deductibles and coinsurance have begun to stabilize, and that they are getting efficient and effective care through the case-management programs, their dissatisfactions will begin to ease—especially if they are also receiving assistance internally from the organization's benefit office, manager, or personnel office.

Internal Communication

Once a decision about plan redesign has been made by the committee, and communicated to and approved by top management, it is time to fully explain the decision to all eligible employees. Committee members should have kept their respective organizations or divisions informed about the ongoing insurance study. Now, as changes are being prepared, small group meetings during which employees learn the details of the plan and why the changes were made should be held. Because not everyone learns in the same manner, it is a good idea to present relevant information using four formats: oral presentations, small discussion groups, written documents, and audiovisual materials. Ideally, the time between the group meetings and implementation of the new benefits plan should be no less than 2 months. However, if this is not possible, there should be at least a 4-week period of time during which employees can be informed about their benefits and allowed to make the necessary choices. This procedure will be explained in greater depth in Chapter 7.

Summary: Initiating Changes

Change is never an easy process. It rarely can be done quickly and effortlessly. The process of changing an organization's medical benefits program underscores the difficulties frequently associated with the change process. If the insurance committee, with the advice and assistance of outside consultants, has determined that a major change is required and that the program should be rebid, the process must be carefully formulated before any action is taken.

Members of the insurance committee have the obligation to keep their fellow employees apprised of the ongoing study and decision-making process. If the committee acts without the support and agreement of the entire organization, the likelihood that the rebidding process will fail increases. Internal communication is an essential component to a successful major change in plan design.

Carriers who wish to bid for the plan designed by the committee and consultants should be willing to give specific examples about how they intend to control costs, manage care, and work with the organization and its insurance committee. If a carrier seems unwilling to do any one of these things, then its commitment to helping control costs must be seriously questioned.

Focus Guide

Research Questions

- Will it be necessary to redesign the medical benefits program, or are there alternatives available to control costs?
- Is your present carrier willing to work with you to design a plan to control rising costs?
- Is your insurance committee knowledgeable about the effects plan redesign may have on the total program?
- Is there an established communication network within the organization that can keep employees informed about potential changes?

Decision Questions

- What is the present time line for studying, suggesting, and implementing changes in the plan design?
- Is your consultant in a position to move forward with your plan? Is he or she able to devote a greater amount of time to your organization?
- Are the individual members of the insurance committee in a position to devote a greater amount of time and attention to this problem?

- Have you identified one senior member of the committee to act as the organization's representative by making appointments for carrier interviews, bid proposal deadlines, and other scheduling issues?
- Have all the available references and data supplied by potential carriers been checked and validated to the satisfaction of the insurance committee?

7
Implementing Changes

Many people mistakenly believe that, once a medical plan has been re-designed and premiums either reduced or stabilized, there is little else to do. If only this were so. In fact, the most challenging part of bringing medical benefit costs under control occurs when an organization begins to implement and maintain the changes.

What Must Be Done Following Plan Redesign

After deciding upon a new program design, a company must take several actions. The funding agreements and the master plan must be finalized with the carrier. Routine meetings between the committee, the carriers, and participating providers should be scheduled. Insurance committee meetings to occur immediately prior to the carrier sessions should be scheduled to allow members to review the periodic reports and prepare questions for the carrier. A process needs to be established for making any needed adjustments to the plan based on data gathered from the carrier, the providers, and staff. Most important, methods for communicating the changes to affected employees should be established. Without all these vehicles in place, the committee's efforts to control costs may prove worthless. Once the plan design changes have been finalized, they should be communicated to covered employees through a plan booklet.

Making Final Agreements with the Carrier

During the bidding process the carriers are only too willing to agree verbally to any special requests you might have. However, once a commitment has been made to a carrier and the time has come to make the agreements final, verbal agreements may suddenly become subject to interpretation. This is why some consultants are reluctant to conduct negotiations with carriers at the end of the bidding process. To minimize these issues, you should (1) have the carriers submit comprehensive written responses, (2) have the complete plan design and funding agreements included in the bid specifications, and (3) make sure that all final negotiations are in writing.

Funding Arrangements

Though the carrier may have been notified, preferably through the consultant, that it is to be awarded the contract, the actual signing of the contract does not occur until all parties are in agreement on its terms and conditions. Most important, all parties concerned should confirm how the premium will be paid for, who will hold the reserves, and who will take the interest on these accounts. If the decision of the insurance committee and the company is to pay for a fully funded program, this decision may be relatively simple. The company will be responsible for paying the full premium, and most likely the carrier will want to hold the interest as it is assuming the total risk.

Minimum Premium Agreements

However, if the committee and the company have opted for a type of self-insured program, the company will benefit most from a minimum premium agreement. Under such an agreement the premium amount necessary to pay medical claims is sent to the carrier on a monthly basis. This amount is typically close to 75 percent of the premium. The carrier will draw on the account as needed, and interest will accrue. It makes financial sense to have the interest retained by the company rather than the carrier. The additional funds can provide for premium stabilization, or a portion can be returned to the operating fund if interest appears to be far in excess of projected needs. It is recommended that the interest be viewed conservatively and saved for premium stabilization, as some premium increases are likely to occur in succeeding years, given current trends. Increases will likely occur even if the program is well managed.

Administrative Charges

In addition to the minimum premium agreement, organizations opting for some form of self-insurance will also be billed for administrative charges on a monthly basis. This amount can range anywhere from 6 to 10 percent of the total premium. It is to the company's advantage to pay administrative fees on a monthly basis even if a 6-month or annual contract is in effect. Remitting monthly allows interest to be earned on the money prior to forwarding it to the plan administrator. Further, small companies operating on a tight cash flow will wish to avoid a large annual cash outlay.

Reserve Accounts

Companies using a self-insured or partially self-insured plan will need to deposit funds into a reserve account. The amount or percentage of premium money that is to go into this reserve account depends on how much money the carrier believes will be needed for premium stabilization, for funding of IBNR, and for the extension-of-benefits (EOB) clause. If the master plan includes a relatively broad-based EOB covering both active and retired employees, the carrier may demand a higher reserve.

Building Reserves.   During the first year of a new plan, the reserve account must be built. Approximately 15 to 25 percent of the total premium should be placed in the reserves, depending on IBNR and the EOB provisions, with interest held by the company rather than the carrier. In subsequent years the reserve can continue to be built as needed. Many carriers at the start of a new contract may want as much as 28 percent placed in reserve. This amount can be negotiated if it appears that a long-term commitment is being made to the carrier, negating the need for a completely funded EOB reserve the first year. Also, with a radically new plan design, it is hard to project IBNR costs. With a good plan design and good cost-management practices, IBNR may turn out to be less than projected by the new carrier.

Reserve as a Percentage of Total Premium.   During the first year of a plan, however, the carrier will prefer to have 25 percent of the total premium directed toward the reserve account. After administrative costs have been paid, this leaves the plan with approximately 65 percent of the premium available to pay medical claims. This funding arrangement will likely guarantee an automatic increase in premium for the following year unless employee usage can be reduced to 65 percent. Since it is unlikely that the insurance committee will be looking for a new carrier in 2 succeeding years, it is generally possible to negotiate with the carrier to keep the reserve amount to 15 to 18 percent.

A sample of a minimum premium agreement and an example of a cash reserve and terminal liability agreement can be found in Appendixes C and D, respectively. In these agreements, the carrier is being held responsible for maximum termination liability under this contract. Should the contract terminate, and the reserves not be large enough to cover IBNR and EOB, the carrier must assume liability. If, however, an employer is willing to assume between 6 and 10 percent of this liability, the amount placed into reserves can be reduced. This assumption of unknown future liability may not be in the best interest of organizations operating on a relatively fixed budget, such as public institutions. However, a private company with large reserves may wish to use a minimum termination liability clause and gamble that costs can be controlled internally, allowing reserves large enough to cover claims submitted following contract termination.

Monthly Statements

As the funding agreements are finalized, the manner in which money is transferred to pay premiums and the form that the monthly statement will take should be addressed. Figure 7-1 is a monthly carrier statement sent by The Insurance Source of the West to Exoskill Manufacturing, a company using a minimum premium agreement. The statement covers the retention or administrative costs associated with the minimum premium agreement. In addition, the employer is placing into a plan benefit account the monthly limit to be used to pay claims. In this case, the employer has not only medical and dental premiums, but also a life and accidental death and dismemberment premium with this particular carrier. The Medicare premium that the employer must pay for all new employees hired after April 1987 is reflected in this statement.

Table 7-1 is a monthly breakdown of the number of Exoskill employees covered under the plan as well as the number of adjustments made to the plan during the month. This total should follow a list of each individual covered under the plan and the type of coverage that individual has. Reports such as these serve as backups to the plan benefit account and may be prepared either by the employer for the carrier or by the carrier for the employer. Depending upon turnover, the size of the company, and the day of the month on which the report is prepared, this report may lag as much as 4 weeks behind actual expenses. Needed adjustments can be made on the following statement.

April 6, 1990

Exoskill Manufacturing
Attn: Gregory Plines
3755 North PCH
Sylmar, CA 91342

Dear Mr. Plines:

For your convenience I have broken down the premium due per
benefit for your April billing statement. I have accounted for all
the adjustments and calculated the reserves separately. I hope
this makes it easier for you to understand your billing statement. If you have any questions or concerns, please don't hesi-
tate to call me at 1-800-555-3542, extension 276.

The breakdown is as follows:

Life premium	$ 3,087.45
Accidental death and dismem- berment (AD&D) premium	$ 1,804.20
PPO premium	$ 30,788.99
Medicare premium	$ 313.55
Dental premium	$ 5,303.09
Total premium	$ 41,297.28
Balance forward	$ −5,001.74
Grand total due	$ 36,295.54
Reserve premiums	
Medical	$ 46,648.56
Dental	$ 7,966.14
Total	$ 54,614.70

Sincerely,

Barbara Harrington
Billing Representative

Figure 7-1. Carrier correspondence.

Table 7-1. Monthly Breakdown of Plan Adjustments for Exoskill
Manufacturing

	Life premium	Medical premium	Medical reserve	Dental premium	Dental reserve	Total premium
Total	3,283.20	33,339.71	50,009.48	5,650.85	8,492.50	100,288.35

2,369 employees:
  1,444 single
  925 with families
259 adjustments:
  202 single employees added
  56 families added
  1 family subtracted

In Table 7-1 the total premium due appears low, given the number of
insureds, because the employer pays only for employees. The carrier receives additional premiums for dependents through premium FSAs
which are directly deposited into the plan benefit account.

Before You Sign the Agreement

Before signing the funding agreements, the employer should carefully
review each component of the agreement. Determining what is covered
under the administrative costs is important. Several pressing questions
may arise, including:

- Do the administrative costs include requested reports?
- Who is responsible for printing and mailing plan design booklets?
- Who is responsible for printing and distributing identification cards?

Preparing the Benefits Booklet

While the funding agreements are being made final, the master contract, which contains all provisions of the policy including plan provisions, eligibility, and funding agreements, should be prepared. Covered
in the master contract is the preparation of the benefits booklet distributed to all covered staff describing the plan provisions and how to file
claims. The booklet should be in a format that can be readily understood by covered employees.

A Realistic Time Line for
Preparation of the Benefits Booklet

Many employers mistakenly believe that a plan booklet can be prepared within a month of the awarding of the contract. While this is not a physical impossibility, it is certainly not prudent to rush the plan book to press. Any mistakes that appear in the booklet distributed to staff will supersede the proposal and responses to the company's requests. This can work to the advantage or the disadvantage of the employer. Some benefits may be listed that shouldn't, or some that should have been included may be left out. A careful review of the master policy and the booklet is often worth the effort. Some carriers will provide a master contract listing plan provisions, funding agreements, and eligibility as well as a separate plan booklet for employees. Unless the plan provisions and plan booklet are identical, problems can arise. Confusion can be minimized by having the plan booklet be a part of the master contract.

Review of the Language Used in the
Benefits Booklet

The review of the plan booklet and the master contract is even more important if the plan design contains unusual features such as carve-out or a 12/12 preexisting limitations clause. Many insurance carriers do not include these features as a routine part of their plans. Therefore, when the master policy is being prepared it is all too easy for someone at the carrier's home office to mistakenly insert more commonly found provisions into the policy.

Good employment practice requires employers to make clear to employees the components of their benefits package. The insurance committee should put considerable effort into working with the carrier to shape the master policy into final form, so that the booklets can be prepared and distributed efficiently. This process can take up to 6 months, which is another reason an employer is advised to start the rebidding process more than 6 months before the end of a contract. In the meantime, employees can be given summaries of benefits and lists of providers to use.

Claims Processors

The carrier's claims office should also have a copy of the employer's plan design and master policy. When processing claims, the claims processors should work from the information contained in the master contract to determine eligibility for claims. Often, claims processors will use the standard company manual unless specifically instructed to use a specific plan design. To effectively assist employees, claims processors will require training in specific plan designs and the methods in which they should be implemented. Having claims processors dedicated to your employees' claims assists with effective implementation. This should be no problem for a group of 500 or more insureds. It is, however, more difficult for smaller companies to persuade carriers to dedicate processors to their claims.

Provision should be made for crediting the employer's account if the claims processors pay submitted claims using the carrier's standard benefits manual rather than claims provisions spelled out in the new plan design. It is advisable for senior staff and members of the insurance committee to meet with representatives of the claims office to review the plan design and the methods that will be employed to pay claims. It would be appropriate at this meeting to stress the importance of maintaining a service orientation in dealing with claimants.

Mistakes in Implementation of the Master Contract

Although the procedures described above may sound overly cautious, it is not uncommon for an employer who is diligent in reviewing claims and working with employees to find that specific plan provisions are not being implemented by the carrier. For this reason, it is crucial for the employer to maintain copies of all contracts, agreements, and letters of understanding between the carrier, consultant, and employer. If an employer does not have the necessary documentation, it will be impossible to have incorrect provisions removed from the plan at renewal time. If the final printing of the master policy and plan booklet do not contain the specifics that were requested in writing at the time of contract signing, the employer's copies of documentation can and should be used during renewal negotiations. This is particularly important in case there may be glaring errors in the booklet which would negate the employer's attempt to control costs.

Western Waves Travel: Dealing with Discrepancies between the Master Contract Language and Actual Practice

Western Waves Tours employs 627 full-time employees and an additional 1500 seasonal employees. Many of Western's employees are older, having retired from their first career and now serving as travel guides around the country. Because of the unusual demographics of its employees, Western sought a 12/12 preexisting limitations clause in the medical benefits program when it changed carriers in 1988. Basically, this provision states that for a 12-month period following initial employment and coverage under the employer's medical benefits program, insureds cannot receive treatment for conditions for which they were treated during the previous 12 months.

The carrier agreed to include this provision in the master contract. However, when claims were processed, eligible employees were subject to the less stringent 3/12 preexisting limitation clause. Had Western not had the carrier's agreement to the 12/12 in writing, it would have been forced to include any claims filed under the 3/12 limitation as part of its experience. With the documentation, Western was able to demonstrate that the carrier was at fault for the incorrect information.

Western gave the carrier two options: (1) to continue with the 3/12 but to count no experience against the renewal for charges incurred by people who should have been covered under a 12/12 or, (2) to immediately implement the 12/12 limitations clause, factoring out of the experience all bills that had been overpaid to date.

Accountability for Carrier Errors

Carriers will often insist that only a few people were overpaid because of mistakes and that the amount is too small to subtract from a company's experience. Insurance carriers need to be reminded that no amount is too small and that ultimately the employer and the employees must fund any premium increases.

Carrier Meetings and Supplied Reports

Once the funding agreements have been concluded, the master policy signed, and the booklets distributed, the insurance committee has a continuing obligation. It should make certain that a smooth cycle of routine meetings with the carriers and the providers has been scheduled. During these meetings, concerned parties should review any problems about the plan design and should monitor expenses both of covered employees and of providers. The same reports that were required during analysis of the plan are needed at this point. A summary of those reports is included in Chapter 5.

If the rebidding included a change in carriers, the format of the reports requested may also have changed. The new carrier should be in a position to interpret the data from the old carrier, drawing comparisons between the old and new programs and making accurate predictions about future costs.

Beginning a New Plan and Carrier

The First 3 Months

As with any new program, the first 3 months of claims experience under the new carrier will not yield accurate data for a number of reasons. During this period, most covered plan participants are in the process of meeting the deductible, decreasing the number of claims that will be filed. In addition, the old carrier is still paying for some costs incurred prior to the end of the contract under IBNR. Further, depending on the EOB clause which was in force with the old carrier, some or all staff who were disabled at the time of the change will be covered under the old carrier. If the new plan offers fewer benefits than the old plan, covered participants will likely have incurred as many of their claims as possible at the end of the old plan so as to avoid using the new plan until necessary.

The conditions noted above, which serve to prevent development of an accurate picture of plan utilization, usually diminish by the fourth month a new plan is in effect. Table 7-2 illustrates a monthly experience summary for an employer that had changed carriers as of January 1, 1989. No claims were issued or cleared during the month of January. However, in subsequent months there was a steady increase in the number of claims filed. The May report begins to give an accurate reflection of monthly experience under the new plan. By that time, issued claims

Table 7-2. Monthly Experience Summary

Experience date	Premium (10%)	Liability (75%)	Issued claims	Cleared claims	Reserve deposit (15%)
1/89	28,814	216,105	0	0	43,221
2/89	28,841	216,308	31,609	11,939	43,262
3/89	32,330	242,475	144,296	149,401	48,495
4/89	30,338	227,535	122,238	116,161	45,507
5/89	28,407	213,053	160,057	155,928	42,614
Total	148,731	1,115,476	458,200	433,429	223,099

Note: Monthly (year-to-date) paid loss ratio—issued claims/liability: 1/89, 0%; 2/89, 7.31%; 3/89, 26.06%; 4/89, 33.04%; 5/89, 41.08% of total premium but 75% of liability.

were running about 75 percent of liability, or the amount being funded each month to cover the claims.

Ongoing Monitoring of Utilization Patterns

Utilization as a Cause of Premium Increase

During a routine meeting with the carrier, the insurance committee was told that a premium increase would probably result the next year if monthly costs edged past 75 percent. After a careful evaluation of the situation, the insurance committee pointed out to the carrier that a different calculation of monthly experience was possible. Rather than following the carrier's calculation formula, the committee took the total of the premium, the liability, and the reserve deposits, and then applied the amount of issued claims against that larger total. Following this formula, claims were actually running at just 56 percent of the amount being funded to the carrier. The committee noted further that the 56 percent, when blended with other issued and cleared claims through January 1989 was actually running at 41 percent. If that 41 percent does not exceed 75 percent at the time of renewal, and can be trended out for another 3 months at that amount, little or no premium increase should be necessary.

When Is Utilization Too High?

It would seem that a carrier with a client experiencing 75 percent utilization should not be concerned. However, carriers often have a perception of the situation that is much different from the client's perception. Carriers will always need approximately 10 percent of the premium for administration costs. Additionally, carriers prefer to keep the reserve as large as possible to offset any potential losses at the end of the plan. Carriers consider it good business practice to hold reserves and return them to the client 12 months following termination. This thinking is reflected in the example above. The carrier felt that 25 percent of the premiums should be used for purposes other than claims. The carrier also preferred a 75 percent utilization of the remaining 75 percent of premium available for claims.

From the employer's standpoint, even with medically wise consumers, costs will probably run at 75 percent of the total premium. If the overall experience does run at approximately 75 percent, even when the first 3 months are deleted and the plan is trended to 12 months based on the 9 months of experience, the employer has a good argument for not increasing premiums. Table 7-2 shows claims experience for Exoskill Manufacturing, the experience of which was shown in Table 1-1. The dramatic drop in utilization can be attributed directly to plan design changes.

Interpreting Coverage Analysis Reports

Table 7-3 shows another type of report that can be used to break down charges. This coverage analysis report provides a breakdown of the total expenses incurred as indicated under the monthly experience summary. The charges listed were close to $1 million during that 5-month period, with actual paid claims running at approximately 50 percent of

Table 7-3. Coverage Analysis Report
January 1, 1989, to May 31, 1989

Code and description	Count	Charges	Paid
01 Hospital room and board	80	$134,949.06	$ 68,159.91
02 Hospital extras	179	139,589.29	103,949.65
03 Ambulance	12	3,126.77	1,926.68
04 Emergency benefits	199	20,058.30	7,661.12
05 Surgery, inpatient	70	58,053.20	27,318.97
06 Surgery, outpatient	333	38,608.10	14,007.52
07 Outpatient surgery expense	204	40,519.18	22,069.13
08 Surgical opinion expenses	1	110.00	110.00
09 Medical care visits	3,414	169,319.05	33,756.58
10 Diagnostic X ray and lab	2,394	89,733.42	30,516.12
11 Misc. major medical expenses	3,158	86,454.23	47,287.33
14 Preventative medical care	178	4,558.00	1,045.84
15 Dental	3,616	203,694.81	117,351.12
16 Special benefits	40	3,075.00	886.20
17 Misc. codes	24	836.71	80.60
Total	13,902	$992,685.12	$476,126.77

Breakdown by coverage	Charges	Paid
Employee	$659,230.30	$304,667.73
Spouse	136,370.07	80,863.51
Dependent	197,084.75	90,595.53
Totals	$992,685.12	$476,126.77

the total due to the impact of deductibles and discounted services through the PPO arrangement. The carrier also provided a breakdown by coverage, which indicated that employees and not their dependents were incurring the highest expenses. This was as it should be since two-thirds of those covered under the plan were employees.

Interpreting Hospitalization Reports

Another report supplied by the carrier focused on hospitalization. This report, Table 7-4, clearly demonstrates the effect plan design changes can have on costs. While the data from the old plan include an average of 5 years of experience, it can be seen that the length of stay was 4.9 days in contrast to the average length of stay of 3.7 days under the new plan for the first 6 months. This data is significant because the conditions that apply to discounting the first 3 months of experience under a new plan are not applicable when considering hospitalization. Most people do not elect to go into the hospital, making the expenses for this type of service consistent from day 1 of a new plan.

While the data discussed in Tables 7-2, 7-3, and 7-4 appear to present a positive picture, they are only an indication that a new plan design has slowed the number of claims incurred. The information contained in reports such as those described above should be forwarded to an insurance consultant for interpretation. It is advisable that an independent consultant be used every 6 months to review the claims experience. The consultant can assist the insurance committee in identifying problem areas in the plan design as well as anticipating increases for the coming year. Since most carriers will not provide an employer with renewal

Table 7-4. Recapitulation of Claims Experience for Exoskill Manufacturing

Hospital Use per 1000 Insureds

	1984	1985	1986	1987	1988	6 months, 1989
Number of admissions	79	91	72	80	80	56.4
Number of days	426	466	301	383	430	211
Average stay (days)	5.4	5.1	4.2	4.8	5.4	3.7

statements until 60 to 90 days prior to termination of the contract, an employer who does not diligently monitor and analyze reports may be in for a shock at renewal.

Investigating Unusual Figures

A final note about reviewing costs. In some instances there appears to be an unusual increase for a particular month. The first thing to check is whether this increase is due to the single catastrophic illness of one employee. If this is the case and everything else is under control, no changes to the plan should be considered. Catastrophic illness expenses can occur in any plan. If the catastrophic case is well managed, the increase in payments should not trigger any premium increase at the time of renewal. Most carriers have a stop-loss policy to protect themselves from losses incurred as the result of catastrophic illness expenses.

Getting the Medical Providers Involved

Providers within the community should also be invited to participate in a review of the plan. If an employer has an indemnity plan that allows employees free access to medical services, provider meetings may be difficult to arrange. However, if the plan is a PPO network, an EPO, or an HMO, provider meetings are much simpler to arrange. Such meetings help to open the channels of communication and let the providers know what the employer and the insurance committee are attempting to accomplish.

The meetings with providers should be used as a vehicle for discussing issues of mutual concern. The committee can make it clear that it is attempting to secure effective and efficient care for employees and their dependents, and that unneeded medical services, unbundling, and code creep are a drain on the plan and will not be tolerated. The doctors can share their perceptions of how the plan is working and offer any suggestions they may have for keeping costs down and providing more effective care.

Dealing with Confidentiality

Some networks of doctors are not comfortable meeting with employers, and they may refuse to meet, on the grounds that meeting might breach the confidentiality of their patients. Employer-provider meetings, however, do not need to violate confidentiality. In reality, most insurance claims forms now contain a waiver-of-information clause which allows a physician to share all pertinent information with the carrier and the organization funding the premium. To ensure that employees do not fear that their medical history will be used in evaluating their performance, a separate agreement can be made with employee groups certifying that this information is to be used only for the monitoring of the plan and not for evaluation or any punitive action against employees. To further safeguard employees' right to privacy, providers can be asked to show the data by number and not by patient. The intent is not to investigate specific employees but rather to pinpoint costs and determine whether they are appropriately managed and paid for.

One topic that should be discussed at all meetings with the carrier and providers is how covered employees are treated when they file claims. It is essential that insureds be treated courteously by claims processors. This is even more critical if plan design changes which shift additional costs onto employees have been made. Replying "Your employer did not choose that benefit for you" is unacceptable—especially when a committee was involved in the design of the plan. The art of saying "no" nicely is an important one for claims processors to learn.

In addition, if claims processors are dedicated to handling claims of your company, your staff can establish some familiarity with the claims office. An employer also finds it advantageous to work with a small group of individuals if issues arise concerning the processing of claims.

This discussion of the process of implementing changes in a medical benefits plan design has been centered on the functions of people outside the employer's organization: the carrier, consultant, and providers. For cost-containment measures to work effectively, however, it is equally important to establish effective internal communication with both individual employees and the organizations that represent them. Success in controlling the cost of an employee benefit program is only as effective as the level of cooperation between employees and management.

Maintaining Exemplary Employee Communication

The insurance committee serves as the centerpiece of the communication process. The committee is in a position to publish the minutes of meetings and to establish effective communication networks. Members of the committee should be chosen from work sites throughout the organization, assuring equal coverage of diverse employee interests. As messengers of the diligent work being conducted on the employees' behalf, the members of the insurance committee will continue to be a valuable resource long after the new plan design has been implemented.

Providing Education Classes

Classes designed to help employees become better medical consumers are also important. Employees should be given the opportunity to learn which questions to ask of their medical providers and how to evaluate the answers. They should come to realize that the process of purchasing medical care is similar to the process of purchasing high-ticket items such as washing machines, cars, or homes. Other topics for classes might include weight control, quitting smoking, stress management, and aerobics and exercise techniques. Although some employers believe that it is up to employees to maintain their health, in actuality a positive approach to health management will help curb medical costs and create a healthier, more productive work force.

Periodic and Regular Information Is Essential

Employees should also receive periodic information from the carrier, the human resources department, or the insurance committee informing them of new trends, modifications in existing programs and policies, and information about classes and notes of interest. This information may be provided in a newsletter, a payroll stuffer, or another employee communication. Figure 7-2 is an example of a payroll stuffer used by an employer who had recently changed carriers.

Meeting with Employees at Their Work Sites

Regular meetings should be held at work sites to discuss insurance and health care concerns with employees. Depending upon the size of the organization and the number of staff members available to perform such services, the meetings can occur quarterly, biannually, or annually. The most important function of these meetings is to help employees understand the employer's concern for their medical well-being. An active employer will make certain that employees understand the various avenues open to them for obtaining further information or help with problems.

If implementation of a new plan design includes a change in carriers,

Please let me introduce myself. I am your employee benefits
manager. I am the person to call for your insurance questions
and concerns. I have been a registered nurse for over 14 years
and have previously worked with two other insurance companies
in the metropolitan area. I am your liaison with the insurance
carrier. I will be providing everyone with a newsletter in August.
In the meantime, here are some tips for the summer.

When going on vacation, remember to take some claims forms
with you. You probably won't need them, but if you do need
medical care, you can ask the hospital to file the claims for you.
Forms can be picked up in the human resources office. Keep in
mind that out-of-area services are counted toward the $250
deductible on the nonpreferred provider side of the network.
You are also responsible for 30 percent of out-of-area charges
plus any charges over the reasonable and customary fees that our
carrier allows.

Are you an expectant parent? Stop into the employee benefits
office to pick up a brochure and information on the services and
free equipment available to our employees.

Figure 7-2. Benefits news bulletin.

effective employee communications becomes even more important.
Written materials must be prepared and meetings held with large
groups of employees, as well as individuals, to explain any benefits design changes. Ideally, employees at each work site will have the opportunity to meet with members of the insurance committee and a representative of the new carrier. Every employee question should be
addressed openly and answered with as much information as possible.
A videotape and a variety of print materials should be left behind at the
work site so that individual employees may refer to them as the need
arises.

Benefits Management Specialist

It is recommended that a benefits management specialist be hired for
the organization. Ideally the person who fills this position should have a
medical background and have as his or her sole function assisting employees and helping to monitor costs. The specialist should also be
someone who has a strong belief in and much experience with managed
care. The purpose is not to encourage employees to spend more money
but to help them to spend their money wisely and to take responsibility
for their health. The benefits management specialist should not be con-

sidered a manager and should not be included in bargaining groups. Independent status will serve to boost employee's confidence in the specialist. Shown in Figure 7-3 is the job description for such an individual.

Figure 7-4 provides questions which might be used by an employer in selecting a benefits management specialist. These questions were prepared in conjunction with an independent consultant and used by representatives of an insurance committee to select a benefits management specialist who had knowledge and background in managed care. Listed under each question in Figure 7-4 are the responses to look for.

Whatever the process used by your company, an effective benefits management specialist will save the employer more than his or her salary by effecting more efficient use of the medical care plan while also helping employees to get the most effective care. An organization without available funds to pay for a benefits management specialist might consider using the savings generated from plan design changes or medical flexible spending accounts to cover this payroll expense.

Flexible Spending Accounts

Staff members should also have the opportunity to meet one on one with representatives of the carrier or with the benefits management specialist to talk about their individual needs. This is essential if a flexible spending account (FSA) is being introduced, or if it is the start of a new year when employees have the opportunity to change their FSAs to keep them in concert with their needs. During an open enrollment period in a company that offers multiple types of coverage, such materials and meetings are equally important. Figure 7-5 provides a memo to all employees of an organization in which radical plan design change was made along with a change in carriers. Appendixes E and F show details of other materials that were used with employees to help them understand the new coverage and the FSAs.

Working with Employees to Decide upon FSAs

When working with employees who are attempting to decide what type of FSA to build, listening to their individual concerns and obligations is absolutely essential. Employees who are paying for dependent care such as child or .elderly parent care, or paying for family premiums, may need help in deciding how to configure their FSAs. Arranging to pay

---

Benefits Management Specialist
Responsibilities

The benefits management specialist will be responsible for educating employees about their benefits, including medical, dental, life, long-term disability, and sick leave. In addition, the specialist's major focus will be to assist employees in becoming better consumers of their benefits. The specialist will perform the following specific duties:

- Orient new employees to the company's benefit philosophy, goals, and specific programs.
- Screen new employees and their dependents for preexisting conditions, and report to the carrier.
- Review employee and dependent eligibility for the medical plan on a regular basis, and report discrepancies to the carrier.
- Provide employees with information on cost-effective providers and fair prices for services.
- Explain benefits plan provisions and claim procedures.
- Initiate and coordinate case management on catastrophic, chronic large claims, and potentially large hospitalizations with the carrier.
- Provide assistance in resolving employee claim disputes.
- Provide information on low-cost, effective health services, free community service programs, and/or other educational programs.
- Interview and counsel long-term disability (LTD) claimants. Work with the carrier, doctors, and staff to return LTD claimants to work as soon as possible.
- Serve as liaison with employer's risk manager to coordinate LTD light-duty program.
- Develop procedures for screening benefits payments and needed referrals to carrier and, as appropriate, staff.
- Prepare information for employees on a variety of topics, including successful hospital confinement, which will assist in helping them become better consumers of health care.
- Review monthly carrier cost-management reports, and prepare analyses. Prepare summary reports on various aspects of the benefits package.

Preferred Qualifications

- Medical or nursing degree or certificate; college background or degree desirable
- Experience working in a medical field, insurance claims office, hospital, or related field for at least 3 to 4 year

---

Figure 7-3. Benefits manager job description.

- Demonstrated ability to manage or establish innovative processes for cost containment and employee education
- Demonstrated ability to understand and analyze new medical technology and carrier cost-containment reports
- Demonstrated ability to work well with others
- Good problem-solving skills
- Demonstrated ability to work well with health care providers
- Demonstrated ability to initiate and follow through on projects with little supervision
- Knowledge of and skills in computers, writing, and group presentation.

WORK YEAR: 12 months

SALARY: $30,000–$35,000

REPORTS TO: Executive director of human resources

TO APPLY: Applicants must submit an application, a résumé, and three current letters of recommendation along with a letter addressing the preferred qualifications.

Figure 7-3. (*Continued*)

for these services with pretax dollars can ease the employee's financial burden as well as freeing additional funds for the employer through reduced contributions to retirement plans and/or FICA. However, once an employee elects to use these plans, further changes cannot be made unless a qualifying event, as prescribed by law, occurs. This makes it imperative that the employee receive the assistance needed to make sound decisions.

Helping Employees to Choose an Insurance Plan

If an employer is offering various types of coverage such as catastrophic care, an indemnity plan, and EPO or PPO networks, it is likely that an open enrollment period will be held annually. When these new plans are introduced, as well as during the open enrollment period, meetings should be held to help employees to decide what changes if any they will make in their current coverage. These changes will range from opting for catastrophic coverage only to opting for the most expensive indemnity plan available.

1. Briefly explain your background and why you are interested in this position.

(Candidate is able to relate his or her background to the job description.)

2. We would like you to respond to a simulation. Please give a 3-minute presentation at one of our work sites introducing yourself, explaining your position, and how you will be able to assist the staff.

(Candidate is able to articulate ideas, understands overall problems.)

3. In relation to the position description for the benefits management specialist, what do you see as the three major strengths you would bring to this position?

(Among candidate's major strengths are strong interpersonal skills, listening skills, organization, ability to work without much supervision, quick to learn, self-directed.)

4. Given this particular position description, what do you see as the major personal skills you would have to work on in order to do this job to your own satisfaction?

(Candidate shows introspection, understanding of self, knowledge of weaknesses and strengths.)

5. Newspapers, magazines, and the media have carried much information concerning the current medical care crisis in this country. Briefly, how would you explain the crisis and the factors contributing to it?

(Candidate understands that the medical care crisis is not one-dimensional and involves not only the consumers but the providers, lawyers, and insurance agents. If the candidate does not have a full grasp of the issue, but does understand that it is not one-dimensional and is able to explain this satisfactorily, that could also be considered positive. Has a broad perspective.)

6. If our organization had limited dollars to spend on medical coverage and a decision had to be made about whether to offer well-baby care or kidney transplants in the plan design, which option would you support the most?

(Candidate understands concepts of cost containment and limited dollars, is able to articulate an argument well, and does not present "a bleeding-heart" syndrome.)

7. An employee calls you and explains that he went to an emergency room during the weekend complaining of severe abdominal pain. As a result, he was given a number of expensive tests, including a chest X ray and blood gasses. The employee is now concerned

Figure 7-4. Benefits manager interview questions.

about the high cost of the visit and wants you to work with the claims office to reduce some of his responsibility for the costs because it was an emergency. How would you respond to this employee?

(Candidate does not have an insurance company mentality, which is often "We won; no change for any reason." Is an employee advocate but not a bleeding heart. Would be able to present appropriate positions to the employee. Would look into the situation with the carrier.)

8. An employee calls to tell you that she has a medical problem which could be resolved with a hysterectomy but for which she will need a monthly Pap smear if a hysterectomy is not performed. The employee's preference is to have the hysterectomy, but the insurance carrier prefers that she continue with the Pap smears until the surgery becomes absolutely necessary. This particular staff member wishes you to call the insurance company convincing it to reverse its decision. How would you approach this situation?

(Candidate adheres to conservative medical practices, understands why surgery would not be called for in this situation, and would assist the employee to understand the alternative and to find ways to live with it.)

9. A manager calls to tell you that one of her staff members appears to have a drinking problem. While the employee does not appear to be under the influence of alcohol on the job, it is clear that the problem does exist and there are times when the employee's judgment is questionable as a result of the problem. What would be your approach to this situation?

(What to look for: appropriate triage skills.)

10.What types of information do you believe an insurance carrier should supply to an employer in order to enable the employer to make good decisions regarding the plan?

(Candidate lists such items as doctor's charges, hospital stays, and analysis of charges.)

11. During your first month of employment, what do you envision as your most important tasks and why?

(Candidate's response shows organizational skills, ability to prioritize, an understanding of the overall situation, and willingness to do quick study.)

12. What questions do you have of us?

(What to look for: the quality of questions asked.)

Figure 7-4. *(Continued)*

November 18, 1988

To: All Employees
From: Human Resources Department Benefits Office
Re: Medical, Dental, Life, and FSA Benefit Coverage

During the past 18 months the insurance committee has been working to contain the rising costs of medical insurance for staff. This work was necessitated by escalating medical costs, overutilization by staff of the medical insurance, and poor controls by the insurance carrier. The work culminated in September with a set of recommendations to change the medical plan design and a decision to rebid for a new insurance carrier.

The rebidding process was concluded on Thursday, November 10, when management approved insurance carriers (IC) as the new medical, dental, life, and flexible spending accounts carrier for Melconi. This decision was reached after days of review, interviewing, and discussion by not only the members of the insurance committee, but also members of all employee bargaining groups and their negotiations team. It is the belief of all of those involved that IC will provide cost-efficient and effective services for the employees of Melconi.

The change to the carrier will require no additional premium costs to the employee or to Melconi for the coverage. The life insurance coverage will continue to be provided at no cost to the employee. The enclosed packet contains the information to help you understand the new coverage and the process you must use to sign up for it. It is imperative that you read all of the materials carefully.

Figure 7-5. Coverage letter from HRD.

Employees Who Want No Coverage

Some employees may wish no coverage for various reasons: they may be financially eccentric, they may feel that they have enough money to cover any catastrophic illness, they may refuse medical care for religious reasons, or they may be covered under another plan. An employer

Attached to this letter you will find:

1. A list of seven meeting dates during which representatives from IC will explain the new coverage. At these meetings you will be given a packet containing names of medical providers and details of the plan.
2. A summary of the medical, dental, and life insurance benefits under the plan.
3. Information on the FSAs.
4. Enrollment forms for the medical, dental, life, and FSA benefits election.
5. Dates when a representative from the carrier will be available in the human resources department to assist employees with enrollment forms and to answer any questions.

The new carrier will be assisting us with the transition and will also help to explain how the new program is to be implemented. We urge you to attend one of the meetings to have your questions answered or to arrange to meet with the carrier's representative in the human resources department.

We hope that you find the transition to be a smooth one.

Remember, all forms are due in HRD prior to December 19.

Figure 7-5 (*Continued*)

should honor such an employee's request if the employee pays for his or her own coverage. In return, the employee should be asked to sign a waiver of coverage. If, however, the employer is paying for the coverage and the reason the employee wants no coverage is because he or she is financially eccentric, a prudent employer will choose to pay for the employee's coverage. Due to risk pooling, it is to the benefit of the employer and employee to have all staff enrolled in a plan being provided at no or little cost to the employer.

Employees Who Want Only Minimal Coverage

Other employees may opt for minimal coverage such as catastrophic only because they are in excellent health and want the larger take-home paycheck that would come with lower premiums. As long as the individual is aware that a catastrophic plan is typically accompanied by very high deductibles and therefore by higher out-of-pocket expenses, this can be a good option for a very healthy individual. Conversely, individuals with extremely high medical needs because of ongoing conditions should probably opt for a more expensive plan offering a wider range of coverage.

Medium Coverage as a Rule of Thumb

The vast majority of an organization's staff members should probably select medium coverage, which may include a PPO network. This choice assures them that they will not have to meet large out-of-pocket expenses and that they have good coverage. Many staff members may select the HMO if this option is available. The most important factor to be taken into account is that each individual has differing medical and financial needs, both of which must be considered in the individual meetings so that proper choices are made.

Once the enrollment period is over and individuals have made their choices, the ongoing communications, classes, and information should be coordinated by the benefits management specialist. The committee should meet bimonthly to review the carrier's reports and the information on staff needs being gathered by the benefits management specialist. In addition, the committee should meet on a biannual basis with the carrier to review all the data.

Through the ongoing work of the benefits management specialist, careful monitoring of claims, and frequent meetings with the carrier and the providers, the employer should be in a strong position to judge whether the plan needs additional modification to control costs or whether it is effective in managing costs.

If the new plan is effective, and staff members have specific requests to enrich the plan, some of these requests can be considered.

Box Creek Land and Cattle Company:
Modifying the Plan to Meet the Unique
Needs of Employees

The Box Creek Land and Cattle Company maintained corporate
offices in Albuquerque, New Mexico. Several hundred employees
and their dependents, however, were scattered on corporate ranches
and real estate developments in Colorado, New Mexico, and
Arizona. When Box Creek implemented a new medical insurance
program, a preferred pharmacy program was included. Employees
who chose to fill their prescriptions at the preferred provider
organization (PPO) pharmacy were billed just $3 per prescription,
regardless of the drug's actual cost.

Initially, there were six PPO pharmacies, all in the Albuquerque
area. While this arrangement proved valuable to employees working
out of the corporate headquarters, it provided no benefits to the
ranch hands and their families, some of whom lived more than 400
miles from the nearest PPO pharmacy.

At the third meeting of the insurance committee, representatives
from the various ranches collectively requested a broader PPO
network. The request was approved by the insurance committee and
forwarded to the carrier. At no increase in plan design cost, the
PPO pharmacy network was expanded to include a pharmacy chain
operating in the Rocky Mountain region. In addition, a small
number of doctors were added to the PPO network to provide ease
of access to employees.

Because the expansion was carried out carefully, there was no
increase in premium cost. Employee trust in the strength of the
insurance committee and Box Creek Land and Cattle Company was
enriched.

Summary: Implementing Changes

Implementing a new plan is not easy. It requires a firm commitment of
time, energy, and patience on the part of senior staff and members of
the insurance committee. As has been discussed, the subject of medical
benefits is both an economic and an emotional issue. Employees naturally will be wary about changes in their benefits plan. They will need
reassurance that they and their families are still covered. They will require education and guidance in selecting the best plan for their particular situation. They will need instruction on how to file claims under
the new plan. All this will require an increased amount of time and energy. If it is done well, however, the initial period of education can result in a net savings down the line.

As a new plan is implemented, it is important to closely monitor the costs and make any needed changes. The employer and its representative insurance committee should never forget that they are the paying customers and that the carrier should be responding to their needs, for data, clarification of claims, or modification of the plan. The carrier and consultants should be assisting the insurance committee in monitoring the impact of federal and state legislation on the plan design and involving employees in any plan changes brought about because of costs requests or legislation. Finally, the board of directors and the CEO must be kept informed about changes in plan design. Only if all the partners work together to continuously improve the plan will the efforts that were made to improve the plan come to fruition.

Focus Guide

Research Questions about the Implementation Process

- Have all the funding agreements been prepared, and are they available for your review and approval?
- Does the master contract reflect all the issues raised during the negotiation period with the new carrier?
- Are the necessary accounts in place for the reserve account?
- Have employees been informed of forthcoming changes to their benefits plan?
- Is the insurance committee in position to facilitate the changes?
- Would the organization benefit from hiring a medical benefits specialist?

Decision Questions about the Implementation Process

- What time schedule has been established for routine delivery of reports to the committee by the new carrier?
- Who will be available to assist employees in completing the paperwork necessary to implement the new plan?
- What are the dates of your open enrollment period?
- Have employees been educated about the FSAs?

8
Planning for the Future

The Kaizen theory of effective management addresses the need for continuous involvement in the process of redesigning and refining the operations of business. The assumption is made that through involvement, the organization can continue to improve its philosophy, operations, and effectiveness. This theory proves to be particularly appropriate when wrestling with the problem of rising medical care costs.

The problems associated with rising health care costs are relatively simple to identify, but difficult to contain. But, using the basic premise of Kaizen and the strategies outlined in this book, the health care benefits manager, in coordination with other members of the organization, can expect to make decisions and initiate actions that will lessen the severity of the problem.

Education: The Focal Point of the Benefits Program

Some of the direct actions an organization must take in controlling rising health care benefit costs include establishment of an insurance committee that represents all facets of the organization, thorough review of all existing and proposed plan designs, and retaining knowledgeable consultants to assist in building a cost-effective medical benefits program. In addition, regular meetings with health professionals, insurance carriers, HMOs, PPOs, utilization managers, and employees should be held. In order for the greatest level of success to be realized, everyone associated with the problem and the solutions must remain informed about any actions taken that will directly affect him or her. Success depends upon the cooperation of all interested parties.

Landmarks of a Successful Cost-Containment Program

A successful cost-containment program must include an ongoing review of diagnosis and prescribed treatments. This requires an effective working relationship with the carrier. Working with the carrier, inpatient care management as well as outpatient ambulatory care management must remain a cornerstone of the health care program. Independent professional utilization managers should be working with the carrier as well as with the organization's benefits management specialist. The goal of this partnership is to assure coordination of services and to assure the success of the shared goal of effective cost management.

Controlling Costs. At present, most efforts to control rising health care benefit costs require reduction of benefits, increase in employee premium contributions, or a combination of both. Whichever step is taken, it will likely result in some erosion of employees' disposable income and possibly in employee loyalty and satisfaction.

   The procedures outlined in this book for analyzing costs and redesigning plans were designed either to minimize premium increases through cost shifting or to keep the established plan intact by increasing premiums. In either instance the process used by the insurance committee to reach the decision should be communicated effectively to the entire employee population in an effort to stave off dissatisfaction.

Employee Communication. In addition to working directly with the carrier and with independent utilization managers, the organization's benefits specialist should take a lead role in making certain that vital employee communication is ongoing. Employee education regarding the type of service they need and what they should expect when seeking a provider should be readily available, and they should know how to gain access to the information.

Employee Education. Although many employees once believed that comprehensive medical and dental care benefits were an entitlement of employment, they are now faced with rapid changes in both the benefits they are provided and the medical profession in general. The benefits specialist should be sensitive to employees' confusion and anxiety while educating them about their new plan or about any changes made in their existing benefits program.

In spite of intensive education and communication, many employees will not understand that benefits are just an alternative use of salary dollars, and part of compensation. They will remain confused about their health care benefits program. And so, the insurance committee, the benefits management specialist, and all those involved with delivery of the medical care benefits must play ongoing roles as educators.

The Future Medical Picture Is Not Bright

There is continuing concern that medical premium increases will continue to negatively affect employees because of the very nature of the health care system in the United States. Evidence shows that significant waste and inefficiency exist in today's health care systems. It is estimated that between 25 and 45 percent of current health care expenditures are unnecessary.

Employees' Responsibility for Managing Utilization

Insurance programs that offer low deductibles have been shown to stimulate use of medical services. Several surveys seem to indicate that individuals who shared in their medical costs (with high deductibles) had significantly less utilization than those who had little or no cost sharing (with low deductibles). Further, heavy consumers of medical services show no significant difference in their health profile over the low users. It appears that efficient care is often more effective than excessive care.

The Need for Strategic Planning

Employers must have strategies which anticipate additional cost increases and which reduce adverse impact on their employees. Appendixes G to K provide examples of such strategic planning. These documents represent the culmination of an intense examination of one public corporation's medical benefits program. The employer had recently changed insurance carriers and significantly altered the benefits plan design in order to curb premiums, which were increasing at a rate of 50 to 60 percent per year.

The models assume that the plan adopted by this employer, which included a choice of PPO or indemnity benefits at the point of access, was working to control costs. The purpose of the models was to provide the insurance committee with information for future decisions about benefits and about adding options for employees.

Even if an employer offers a variety of options to employees, models such as those shown in the appendixes and the discussion of their impact serve to clarify how various plan designs can have an impact on premium costs.

It is not enough for employers and employees to be concerned only with their own medical benefits plan. Many outside influences affecting carriers, consultants, employers, and providers can disrupt the most carefully thought out and implemented plan.

Involvement Is Crucial

Employers need to become involved in reviewing potential legislation and ethical issues that affect medical care. Through local, state, and federal lobbying agencies, they need to analyze the impact of proposed mandated care, to assist in promoting that which is essential to the welfare of individuals, and to work to limit or defeat nonessential services, such as providing hairpieces to people who become bald because of rare diseases.

Most individuals who are knowledgeable about medical care coverage believe that some form of mandated health care coverage for all individuals is inevitable. However, in countries with mandated health care coverage, there appear to be two systems of health care providers existing side by side: one which covers everyone and one for those who can pay for more personalized service. If a basic floor of coverage that all employers must offer to all employees were set, two-thirds of the current uninsured would be covered, alleviating the necessity of a mandated program for all. Employers and employees are already paying for a mandated program through subsidy of indigent care. Limiting the scope of such a program makes more choices available to individuals, and concurrently places more responsibility on them for maintaining their health and selecting necessary services. Further, if this limitation of scope could be achieved, greater efforts could then be made to extend coverage to uninsureds.

There are also proposals for layering health care by age, providing more services for younger people and slowly tapering these services off as individuals age. We are a maturing population. By the year 2010, 6 working people rather than the current 16 will be supporting retirees. In this context, layering health care becomes an issue of great significance.

The Ethics of Medical Benefits

Additionally, increased focus on health care benefits will precipitate deeper examination of many ethical issues that surround modern medical practice. Already, several carriers and organizations are grappling with plan designs in which prenatal and well-baby care is taking precedence over transplant surgeries. Research indicates that prenatal care can result in healthier babies and that well-baby care during the first 2 years of a child's life can offset future illnesses. However enlightened these policies may be, they are still difficult for the parent of a 5-year-old child who needs a liver transplant to understand.

There is still an ongoing debate about the appropriateness and use of extraordinary medical treatment. Insurance carriers, employers, and physicians must ask themselves and their patients whether society is in a position to expend millions of dollars each year for extraordinary health care that may prolong, but not assure, life. Other issues, such as mandated care, infant intensive care, and organ transplants, will likely be debated in the months and years to come. There is every indication that these and other debates will continue for some time to come because, at present, there are no clear answers. What is evident is that there are no panaceas.

Until every individual who is a part of the current health care crisis—employers, employees, carriers, providers, and lawyers—takes responsibility for part of the problem, it will not be solved. The concepts and actions described in this book should bring the solution a bit closer to reality.

Postscript

Throughout this book reference has been made to plan design changes that were designed by one employer's insurance committee and implemented the following year. During the year following implementation, both usage and costs were contained. While other businesses in the area were faced with a 20 to 30 percent increase in premiums, this employer saw just an 11 percent increase in premiums.

However, following the departure of several key personnel in senior management as well as a large state reduction in financial support, benefits management and design became less important than job security. Energy which had been directed to employee education about medical benefits was diverted to address negotiations and potential layoffs. While this situation is understandable, it only underscores the need to continue with the education of employees and to remove benefits from an area of negotiation and place them where they belong: as the focus of a common problem with a common solution.

The number of providers in the plan was allowed to increase. Costs began to rise as case management became more difficult. The familiar problems of code creep and overuse of the plan began to show up. Like many neighboring business organizations, this employer can certainly expect to see health care benefits costs rise in the near future.

This situation is being repeated again and again throughout the country. Employees who are accustomed to having their entire health care benefits package paid by the employer are willing to stage walk-outs, strikes, and work stoppages to maintain this level of health care benefits. While such employee strategies may prove effective in the short run, they are certain to promote a further weakening of this country's health care system. Rather, a collaborative effort to solve the problem is needed. Employers and employees must work together to seek solutions. Trust must be built, monitored, and sustained.

Employers and employees simply cannot afford to meet the annual double-digit premium increases. At some point, unless changes are made, the system will deteriorate so far that only a national health care system will seem effective. However, as has been demonstrated in other countries, a national health care system leads to a two-tiered system of medical services: one level of treatment and service for those who can afford to pay the bills, and a lower tier for those who must rely on na-tionalized medicine for service. A system that provides universal cover-age but does not require initiation of a national health care policy for all but the unemployed and uninsured should be the goal of everyone in-volved in the problem of rising health care costs. This implies that the focus of the national health care policy should be on the unemployed and uninsured.

One effective way of avoiding this continued decline is to encourage all segments of the organization to get involved in solving the problem before an arbitrary solution is imposed by Congress, the same people who brought us Medicare and social security.

Letter of Agreement for Consulting Services

March 19, 1989

Rebecca S. Simonson-Donnoly
Executive Director of Human Resources
Cable-45 Telecommunications Corporation
P.O. Drawer K
Caldicott, New Hampshire

Re: Consulting Services

Dear Rebecca:

As a follow-up to our previous correspondence outlining the consulting and actuarial services which we are prepared to render to Cable-45 and the recent meeting which we had, we have prepared this revised letter of services for your review and comment. As you know, employee benefits plans are subject to both federal and state legislation and regulation. These laws and regulations affect plan provisions, levels of benefits, nondiscrimination requirements, monitoring of plan agreements, record keeping, claims processing and payment, participant appeals and rights, communications with employees, and continuation provisions.

While our services encompass a broad range of expertise, we do not, as you know, provide legal, administrative, or claims processing services. It is within this framework that we set forth the ongoing regular services that we will provide to your company and an estimate of the fees for such services.

General Consultation

As consultant and actuaries for Cable-45, we provide the ongoing regular services summarized below:

1. Consultation. We will be available for consultation on any aspects of the benefits plans, including claims, reserves, and insurance company performance, as well as the plan's overall progress and development.

We will be available to your staff for consultation on changes in the benefits plan and in eligibility, underwriting provisions, administration, and other relevant matters.

2. Annual report. We will prepare for you an annual report analyzing claims experience, benefits paid, contributions, administrative expenses, gross and net cost of insured benefits, new cost of any insured coverages, and other relevant aspects of the plan.

This report includes a projected income and expense budget based on an analysis of prior experience and known or anticipated factors affecting future operations. Together with an evaluation of the plan's reserve position, this budget serves as a guide to financial and benefits planning decisions.

3. Benefit changes. We will provide advice and then take appropriate action as authorized by the human resources department to implement any benefit changes including revision in premium and plan record-keeping procedures, master policy certificates, and booklet amendments or modifications.

4. Insurance company negotiations. As authorized by Cable-45's human resources department, we will negotiate with the insurance companies to obtain appropriate rate adjustments. If an insurance company's proposed annual retention is not consistent with its projections, or if the renewal premium rates do not appear justified by claims experience, we will attempt to obtain more favorable results for Cable-45.

5. Organization of issues. We shall be available for consultation and shall assist in preparing meeting agendas to aid Cable-45 in reaching decisions about issues that arise in the course of operation; in response to our annual report, plan design, or administrative questions; or in connection with national or industry trends or public policy.

6. Administrative support. We shall continue to be available for consultation with Cable-45, as requested, with regard to routine changes in forms and procedures and general record keeping, in terms of efficiency and cost. It is noted that compliance with the record-keeping requirements of laws or regulations is subject to the advice of legal counsel. However, we also shall be available for consultation in this regard, from a nonlegal standpoint.

7. Trends in legislation, new benefits, plan design. By means of our periodic newsletter and special advisory reports, we

shall continue to keep you apprised of new developments in
the employee benefits field that may bear upon your planning and policy decisions. However, specific technical compliance with new legislation or regulations that occur after
the effective date of this retainer generally will be treated as
supplementary service, at an additional fee, based on our regular time charge rates.

We will, as appropriate, coordinate our efforts with those of
Cable-45, insurance carriers, and other benefits providers.

We will continue to attend insurance committee meetings
and meetings with Cable-45 personnel, as appropriate. We
anticipate approximately 8 to 10 such meetings each year to
provide the above services.

In consideration of these general ongoing services, our annual fee will be $6000.

Specific Consultation

Request for Personnel

If Cable-45 instructs us to secure bids for underwriting the benefits programs, we will prepare and send a detailed specifications letter to a number of insurance companies of Cable-45's
choosing. The specifications letter will place special emphasis
on such items as:

1. Exact benefits to be provided
2. Gross premium rates
3. Net premium rates
4. Insurance company reserve practices
5. Master contract provisions
6. Retention
7. Answers to specific questions
8. Claims utilization information and frequency of reports
9. Cost-management programs
10. Claims processing facilities, practices, and assistance
11. Benefits provider arrangements
12. Data analysis
13. Employee communications and educational materials

We will provide a written analysis of proposals received in a
comparative type format to include the above items.

Once Cable-45 has selected an insurance carrier or carriers to
underwrite all or a portion of the benefits programs, we will in-

struct the carrier or carriers to submit draft copies of their master policy or policies, which we will review and analyze in their entirety in order to make certain that they are in compliance with the specifications letter and the proposal. Our services will also include review of summary plan descriptions for the new carrier or carriers.

Our fee to provide these services will depend on the coverages for which proposals are requested. If proposals were requested for life insurance, accidental death and dismemberment, dental and medical, our fee would be in the range of $4000 to $6000.

If proposals were requested for long-term disability, our fee to perform the above services would be in the range of $1500 to $2500.

Tax-Sheltered Annuity Program

1. We will assist in the drafting of general guidelines that must be met by providers prior to their being approved to solicit tax-sheltered annuities. In addition, we will assist in an annual review of those guidelines to assure that they are kept current and appropriate.

2. When instructed by Cable-45, we will secure competitive proposals from providers. (Competitive bids should be secured not more than once per year, preferably on a biannual basis.)

3. We will prepare a written analysis of all proposals submitted by the various providers for Cable-45's consideration.

4. We will assist in the review of administrative procedures required by the providers to make certain they conform to those stipulated by Cable-45.

Our fee to provide these services would be in the range of $2500 to $3500, based on proposals being requested not more than biannually.

Claims Utilization Analysis

Working in conjunction with Cable-45 and the insurance carrier or carriers, we will establish reporting requirements and format to the satisfaction of Cable-45. The reports will be condensed to effective management reports on varying frequencies, i.e., quarterly summaries, a more detailed semiannual report, and a comprehensive annual report. These reports will be in addition to monthly reports provided by the insurance carrier or carriers and will provide comparisons with previous time periods and applicable norms.

Our annual fee to provide these services will be based on our actual time charges, not to exceed $3000.

Other Services

The above consulting services do not catalog all the detailed matters which may arise during the course of your benefits program's annual operation that require consulting services. Also, it is difficult to predict in advance whether your benefits program will be involved in long, complicated, time-consuming special problems, and if so, to what extent.

If our assistance involves services which are beyond, but incidental to, the aforementioned services, we will render such services within the scope of each listed service. If, on the other hand, the occasion requires the expenditure of time not anticipated in the retainer, we will proceed only after consultation with Cable-45 about services and fees.

In addition to the items referred to earlier, some further supplementary consulting services which may be required by Cable-45 are listed below.

* Detailed analysis of and compliance with new legislation or regulations. Examples include COBRA and Section 89 antidiscrimination provisions.
* Litigation or lawsuits.
* Comprehensive plan redesign or cost restructuring.
* Negotiations with providers regarding specific discount arrangements.
* Any services not specifically set forth in the retainer.

The above services are not freestanding, with the exception of general consultation. Any of the other services would require at least a retainer.

Sincerely,

Raymond J. Irwin

Appendix **B**

Employee Benefits Needs Survey

Benefits Keep Getting More Expensive and More Important!

The survey is introduced to the employees by a letter that summarizes the effects of increasing medical costs on the company and on employees (Figure B-1).

Dear Employee:

What is the fastest-growing area of company expense? Employee benefits. The reason is skyrocketing health care costs for employees and their dependents.

How big is the problem? This year, our employees and their dependents will spend nearly $4.2 million on health care benefits, up 30 percent from last year.

The effects of medical care inflation are evident. In the past few months, benefits have had to be reduced, and premiums you pay for your dependents' health care coverage have risen. Further changes may be necessary to balance needed coverage and cost.

For these reasons, we are conducting a thorough review of the benefits programs, and your input is vital. By completing this survey, you can tell us what you think of the current benefits and what your priorities are for covering health care services and getting needed financial protection.

The survey should take 10 to 15 minutes to complete. If you have any questions, please call the human resources department.

Figure B-1.

Health Care Survey

What do you think? What would be the best benefits arrangement for you?

Here is your opportunity to tell us.

Instructions

Read each question carefully. Choose the response that best represents your answer or point of view. For most questions, you can simply circle the number that precedes your answer. Special instructions are given for some questions. In these cases, please follow the instructions carefully.

Health Care Costs

1. Your compensation includes your pay *and* the amount the company spends on your benefits. How important are employee benefits to you?
   1 Very important
   2 Somewhat important
   3 Somewhat unimportant
   4 Not important at all
   5 Not sure

2. How much do you think the company pays toward your benefits every year?
   1 Less than $250 an employee
   2 $250, but less than $500 per employee
   3 $500, but less than $750 per employee
   4 $740 but less than $1000 per employee
   5 More than $1000 per employee

3. The company's insurance pays a portion of medical and dental costs. You pay a portion in the form of deductibles and copays. How acceptable is your share of the costs?
   1 Very acceptable
   2 Somewhat acceptable
   3 Somewhat unacceptable
   4 Very unacceptable
   5 Not sure

4. How much did you and your covered family members spend on medical and dental care in 1987? (Please ignore any premiums you paid for dependents or any amounts you were paid by insurance.)
   1 Less than $250

2   $250, but less than $500
3   $500, but less than $750
4   $740 but less than $1,000
5   More than $1000

5. If you could choose how much of your compensation would go toward benefits, what is the maximum you would spend on benefits per year?
1   Less than $500 per year
2   More than $500 but less than $1000 per year
3   More than $1000 but less than $2000 per year
4   More than $2000 but less than $3000 per year
5   More than $3000

6. Given a choice among compensation plans that would cost the company the same amount of money it currently spends, would you prefer:
1   The same pay and same benefits
2   More take-home pay and lesser benefits
3   More benefits and less take-home pay

Covered Expenses

Even if it meant having to pay for the benefit yourself or reducing another benefit, how do you feel about the items listed below? If you would *improve* the benefit, circle the number 1. If you would *reduce* the benefit, circle 2. If you would *leave the benefit the same,* circle 3.

Medical Coverage

7. Routine office calls, tests, and minor treatment	1	2	3
8. Hospital or surgical care	1	2	3
9. Maternity, prenatal care	1	2	3
10. Pediatric care	1	2	3
11. Catastrophic accident or illness care	1	2	3
12. Long-term nursing or custodial care	1	2	3
13. Prescription drugs	1	2	3
14. Medical equipment	1	2	3
15. Emergency care	1	2	3
16. Mental health care	1	2	3

17. Chiropractors	1	2	3
18. Drug or alcohol use rehabilitation	1	2	3

Dental Benefits

19. Routine, preventive care	1	2	3
20. Major work such as crowns, bridges	1	2	3
21. Orthodontic care	1	2	3

Vision Care Benefits

22. Routine care	1	2	3

Hearing Care Benefits

23. Routine care	1	2	3

Day-Care Benefits

24. Routine care	1	2	3

25. Do you have too much coverage for some expenses and not enough for others?

 1 Yes
 2 No
 3 Not sure

From the list below, choose the three most important benefits changes the company could make. Write the numbers here:

26. Most important   ____

27. Second most important ____

28. Third most important   ____

 1 Maintain current benefit levels, even if it reduces future pay increases.
 2 Lower premium costs for dependents.
 3 Increase deductibles and copayments to control costs.
 4 Lower deductibles and copayments, even if it reduces future pay increases.

5   Lower benefits paid by the medical plan for routine care, to reduce costs.

6   Lower benefits paid by the medical plan for catastrophic care, to reduce costs.

7   Lower benefits paid by the dental plan, to reduce costs.

8   Offer a "cafeteria-type" or flexible benefits plan that would allow employees to choose between benefits and pay dollars.

29. Considering what you know about benefits offered by other companies, rate our benefits program:

1   Excellent
2   Fairly good
3   Average
4   Not very good
5   Poor
6   Don't know what other companies offer

30. Rank the following benefits in order of importance to you (1 is most important):

Dental   ____
Disability   ____
Medical   ____
Life insurance ____

For the questions below, circle the number 1 if you choose the response *very important,* 2 if *somewhat important,* 3 if *somewhat unimportant,* or 4 if *not at all important.*

31. How important were benefits in your   1   2   3   4
    decision to work here?

32. How important is the level of your take-   1   2   3   4
    home pay in your decision to remain
    working here?

33. How important is it to you to have   1   2   3   4
    more freedom than you now have to
    choose your benefits package?

Circle 1 for *yes,* 2 for *no,* or 3 for *not sure.*

34. Should length of service be a factor in   1   2   3
    determining how much employees pay
    for their insurance?

35. Should different premiums be charged   1   2   3
    to employees depending on their use of
    health care services?

36. Should frequent or continual users of   1   2   3
health care services have higher payroll
deductions and/or greater out-of-pocket
costs than occasional low users?

37. If you could buy additional life insurance through the company, would you?

38. If you could buy life insurance for your spouse and dependent children, would you?
 1 Yes
 2 No
 3 No dependents
 4 Not sure

39. The number of paid sick days provided by the employer is
 1 Very adequate
 2 Adequate
 3 Somewhat inadequate
 4 Very inadequate
 5 Not sure

40. The company's long-term disability plan guarantees 60 percent of
your gross income if you become totally disabled. Do you consider these
benefits
 1 Very adequate
 2 Adequate
 3 Somewhat inadequate
 4 Very inadequate
 5 Not sure

41. Would you be willing to join a health plan (HMO or PPO) which required you to use specific physicians and hospitals?
 1 Yes, if the costs were less
 2 Yes, if the benefits were better
 3 No
 4 Not sure

Insurance Company Service

42. If you had one or more medical or dental claims in the past year,
were they processed to your satisfaction by the insurance company?
 1 Yes
 2 No
 3 Never had a claim (*Skip to 44.*)

43. Was information about your claim readily available?
   1 Yes
   2 No
   3 Didn't have a question (*Skip to 45.*)

44. Was the information you received accurate?
   1 Yes
   2 No
   3 Not sure

45. How good a job does the employer do of keeping you informed about benefits?
   1 Poor
   2 Fair
   3 Good
   4 Excellent

From which of the following sources do you get benefits information? (*Check all that apply.*)

46. Program booklets   ____

47. Human resources   ____

48. Immediate supervisor   ____

49. Biweekly company newsletter   ____

50. Bulletin board notices   ____

51. Employee meetings   ____

52. Other employees or "grapevine"   ____

Access to Health Care Services

53. Which of the following cities is nearest to where you normally seek medical care?
   1 Chicago
   2 Elk Grove
   3 Aurora
   4 Evanston
   5 Hinsdale

54. Are you satisfied that you could get medical care quickly in an emergency?
   1 Very satisfied
   2 Somewhat satisfied
   3 Somewhat dissatisfied

4   Very dissatisfied
5   Unsure

Circle 1 if your response is *excellent,* 2 if *good,* 3 if *fair,* 4 if *poor,* 5 if *not sure.*

55. In your opinion, what is your current health status? 1 2 3 4 5

56. In your opinion, what is your family's health status? 1 2 3 4 5

If you see a doctor *never or rarely,* circle 1; if *at least once a year,* circle 2; if *two or three times a year,* circle 3. If you are *under ongoing care,* circle 4; of if you are *seriously ill,* circle 5. If none of the above describes your situation, circle 6.

57. Which of the statements above most closely describes your own use of medical services? 1 2 3 4 5 6

58. If you cover your family on your benefits plan, which statement most closely describes their use? 1 2 3 4 5 6

For each question below, circle 1 if you were *very satisfied,* 2 if you were *somewhat satisfied,* 3 if you were *somewhat dissatisfied,* or 4 if you were *very* dissatisfied. If none of the above describes your reaction, circle 5.

59. Overall, how do you feel about the health care services you and your family have received in the last few years? 1 2 3 4 5

60. How did you feel the last few times you saw a doctor? 1 2 3 4 5

61. Was your doctor a PPO doctor?
   1 Yes
   2 No
   3 Don't know

When you or a member of your family needs a doctor, what factors influence your decision to use a particular doctor? From the nine factors in the list, choose the three that are most important to you, and write the numbers here:

62. Most important   ____

63. Second most important   ____

64. Third most important ____
1 Experience, reputation in the medical community, credentials
2 Personal convenience—office location, hours, availability of appointments
3 Familiarity with your medical history
4 Personal manner, attitude, time spent listening and taking you seriously
5 Ability to answer your questions in understandable terms
6 Availability to discuss your problems if you need help
7 Reasonable fees for service
8 Ability to diagnose problem and prescribe effective treatment
9 Provision of information on how to avoid problems and enjoy good health in the future

Choose the three factors that would have most influence upon your decision to use a particular hospital, if you needed to go to a hospital. Write the numbers here.

65. Most important ____

66. Second most important ____

67. Third most important ____
1 Doctors on staff
2 Treatment by nursing staff
3 Cost of care
4 How long you must stay in the hospital
5 Use of latest medical equipment
6 Rooms or other facilities
7 Location, personal convenience
8 Reputation within the community for quality care

68. Have you or a member of your family stayed overnight in a hospital in the last year?
1 Yes
2 No (*Skip to question 71.*)

69. Who decided which hospital to use?
1 N/A
2 The doctor
3 You or a member of your family
4 Someone other than a member of your family

70. Considering the cause of hospitalization, do you think the time spent in the hospital was
1 Too long
2 Too short
3 About right

4   Not sure

71. What items would you like to have covered by the benefits program that aren't now covered? List them here.

_____

_____
_____
_____
_____

72. Do you have any other concerns about your benefits program that you would like to communicate? List them here:

_____

_____
_____
_____
_____

Profile Information

73. What is your age?
    1   Under 30
    2   30–39
    3   40–49
    4   50–59
    5   60 or above

74. What is your gender?
    1   Female
    2   Male

75. How many years have you worked for the company?
    1   Less than 2 years
    2   2–5 years
    3   6–10 years
    4   11–20 years
    5   More than 20 years

76. How much do you work?
    1   Full-time
    2   Part-time, less than 20 hours per week
    3   Part-time, more than 20 hours per week

77. Which best describes your status as a wage earner?
    1   Sole wage earner with one job
    2   Sole wage earner with multiple sources of support (such as two jobs)
    3   Primary wage earner in family with two or more incomes
    4   Secondary wage earner in family with two or more incomes

78. Do you have another medical insurance plan available to you?
    1 Yes
    2 No
    3 Don't know

79. Does your spouse work for the company?
    1 Yes
    2 No

80. Which of these cities is nearest to where you live?
    1 Chicago
    2 Elk Grove
    3 Aurora
    4 Evanston
    5 Hinsdale

81. How many people (children and adults, including yourself) do you cover under the benefits plan? Write the answer here:____

82. What is your total family income?
    1 Less than $20,000
    2 $20,000–$30,000
    3 $30,001–$40,000
    4 $40,001–$50,000
    5 $50,001–$60,000
    6 More than $60,000

Do not sign your name.
Your responses will be kept confidential.
Thanks for participating.

Appendix C
Minimum Premium Agreement

This Minimum Premium Agreement, effective February 1, 1986, is between Davison, Donohue, and Wexler (Employer) and Insurance Carriers, Ltd. (Carrier).

WHEREAS, Employer has established an ERISA plan (Plan) of health and welfare coverage for certain employees; and

WHEREAS, the majority of the Plan *health* coverage is self-insured by Employer and the remainder insured by Carrier under Group Policy GPZ-1022; the majority of the Plan *dental* coverage is self-insured by employer and the remainder under Group Policy GPD-Z1022 [Policy(ies)]; and

WHEREAS, the Policies expressly assume liability only for Plan coverage in excess of the self-insured Plan liability of the Employer;

THEREFORE, IN CONSIDERATION of the following promises, Carrier and Employer agree as follows:

Definitions

"Intrastate First" shall mean the Intrastate Bank of Glenwood, Glenwood Springs, CO.

"Plan Benefit Account" shall mean the Intrastate First bank account on which self-insured Plan benefit payment drafts are drawn.

"Transfer Bank" shall mean the bank selected by Employer and approved by Carrier.

"Monthly Liability Limit" shall mean the aggregate of an amount determined each month by multiplying the number of employees covered under the health Plan during the preceding month in each of the following classes by the amounts listed below.

GPZ-1022

Class 1	Amount
Employee	$ 43.91
Employee and spouse	118.69
Employee, spouse, and child(ren)	155.29
Employee and child(ren)	80.53

Class 3	Amount
Employee	$ 42.80
Employee and spouse	116.03
Employee, spouse, and child(ren)	152.61
Employee and child(ren)	79.38

GPD-Z1022

	Amount
Employee	$11.74
Employee and spouse	23.47
Employee, spouse, and child(ren)	33.68
Employee and child(ren)	21.95

"Transfer Account" shall mean the Transfer Bank account in which Employer deposits the Monthly Liability Limit.

"Transfer Amount" shall mean the periodic transfer of funds required to maintain the Plan Benefit Account at a minimum daily balance of $20,000.

"Special Transfer Amount" shall mean the portion of any funds available to reimburse Carrier for Plan payments made under their Policy(ies) during periods when such funds were not available from the Transfer Account or to satisfy Carrier's terminal liability.

"Annual Liability Limit" shall mean the sum of all monthly Liability Limits each Policy year, or if the Policy(ies) terminate(s) during the policy year, the number of months the Policy(ies) was (were) in force during the Policy year.

1. Employer's Responsibility
    1.1   The Plan Benefit Account shall be established in the Employer's name at Intrastate First.
    1.1.1   Employer shall not be required to pay any charges made by Intrastate First in connection with the Plan Benefit Ac-

count, provided all the terms of this Agreement are met by Employer.

1.1.2 Employer shall not be entitled to any interest on the Plan Benefit Account

1.2 On or before February 1, 1986, Employer shall deposit the Transfer Amount in the Plan Benefit Account.

1.3 On or before February 1, 1986, Employer shall establish the Transfer Account in the Transfer Bank.

1.3.1 Employer shall pay any charges made by the Transfer Bank in connection with the Transfer Account.

1.3.2 Employer shall not be entitled to withdraw from the Transfer Account except:

1.3.2.1 For any interest payable on the Transfer Account; and

1.3.2.2 As provided for by the terms of this Agreement.

1.4 On or before February 1, 1986, and by the first business day of each calendar month thereafter, Employer shall deposit the Monthly Liability limit in the Transfer Account.

1.5 No later than the first business day of each calendar month commencing February 1, 1986, Employer shall notify Carrier of the amount of the deposit to the Transfer Account and shall mail to Carrier at the Home Office an exhibit reflecting the calculation of the preceding month's Monthly Liability limit.

1.6 Employer shall require the Transfer Bank to:

1.6.1 Wire transfer the Transfer Amount to the Plan Benefit Account at Intrastate First immediately following Carrier's request.

1.6.2 Mail a check for any Special Transfer Amount to Carrier, immediately following Carrier's phone request.

1.6.3 Acknowledge in writing to Carrier that the Transfer Bank has a copy of and will act in accord with the terms of this Agreement with respect to the provisions relating to the Transfer Account.

1.7 Employer shall send or arrange to transit any Special Transfer Amount directly to Carrier immediately following Carrier's telephone request.

1.8 Employer shall not make or authorize any account transaction not specifically provided for in this Agreement without the written authorization of Carrier.

1.9 Employer agrees that self-insured Plan coverage shall be the same as insured Plan coverage under the Policy(ies), but that coverage under the Policy(ies) is in excess of self-insured Plan coverage.

1.10 Employer shall make available for Carrier's inspection, at any reasonable time during the continuance of this Agreement and within 1 year thereafter, Employer's books and records which may have a bearing on this Agreement.

1.11 Employer shall indemnify and hold Carrier harmless against any and all loss, damage and expense, including attorneys' fees, resulting from or arising out of:

1.11.1   Any taxes assessed against or paid by Carrier in connection with self-insured Plan coverage;
1.11.2   Any loss, liability, damage or expense or other cost or obligation resulting from any claim, assessment, demand or lawsuit against Carrier in connection with self-insured Plan coverage; or
1.11.3   Employer's failure to provide appropriate notice to all Plan participants that Employer is liable for payment of the self-insured Plan coverage and that this portion of the Plan is not insured by Carrier.

2. Carrier's Responsibilities

2.1   Carrier shall instruct Intrastate First to notify the Transfer Bank to wire Transfer Amount as required to maintain the Plan Benefit Account at minimum daily balance of $20,000.
2.2   Carrier may ask Employer to send or arrange to transmit any Special Transfer Amount directly to Carrier:
2.2.1   To reimburse Carrier for payments made under the Policy which were Employer's liability under the self-insured portion of the Plan;
2.2.2   To reimburse Carrier for any deficits incurred with respect to the Policy; to satisfy Carrier's Policy terminal liability.
2.3   Carrier shall not request any Special Transfer Amount funds in excess of funds authorized in Provision 2.2 above.
2.4   Carrier shall perform all administrative functions necessary for the proper maintenance of the Plan Benefit Account, including:
2.4.1   A monthly reconciliation of the Plan Benefit Account bank statement;
2.4.2   An annual accounting of both the Plan Benefit Account and the experience under the Policy.
2.5   Carrier shall not make or authorize any account transaction not specifically provided for in this Agreement without the written authorization of Employer.
2.6   Carrier shall provide the following claims administration for the self-insured portion of the Plan:
2.6.1   Furnish personnel, establish claim handling procedures and provide claims-handling facilities.
2.6.2   Process claims in accord with ERISA standards and with Plan coverage.
2.6.3   Issue all Plan benefit payments on Plan Benefit Account drafts.
2.6.4   Bond all Carrier employees who handle monies or property of the Employer in an amount not less than $250,000.
2.7   Carrier shall not be responsible for Employer's compliance with the requirements of ERISA or any state or federal laws affecting self-insured coverages, but Carrier will cooperate in coordinating self-insured and insured coverage under the Plan for ERISA reporting purposes.

3. Plan Liability
    3.1   Employer shall be liable under the self-insured portion of the Plan for all Plan coverage not to exceed the Annual Liability Limit. Carrier shall be liable under the Policy only for Plan coverage in excess of the Annual Liability Limit.

4. Assignment
    4.1   No assignment by either Employer or Carrier pertaining to this Agreement shall be valid without the written consent of the other party.

5. Applicable Law
    5.1   This Agreement shall be governed by the laws of the state of Colorado.

6. Termination
    6.1   This Agreement shall be automatically terminated upon the earliest of:
        6.1.1   The date the Policy(ies) terminate(s)
        6.1.2   Any date mutually agreed upon between Carrier and Employer
        6.1.3   The date Employer fails to deposit the monthly Liability Limit in their Transfer Account
        6.1.4   The date the Employer withdraws the authorization to Transfer Bank to wire transfer fund to the Plan Benefit Account
        6.1.5   The date the Plan is terminated by law
    6.2   Carrier may terminate this Agreement on any renewal date of the Policy(ies) provided Carrier gives Employer one month's advance written notice.

7. Annual Accounting
    7.1   Following any annual Policy accounting or following the final accounting after termination of the Policy(ies):
        7.1.1   Carrier shall reimburse Employer for any Plan payments Employer may have made which were the obligation of Carrier; or
        7.1.2   Employer shall reimburse Carrier for any Plan payments or expenses incurred by Carrier which were the obligation of Employer according to the terms of this Agreement.

DAVISON, DONOHUE, AND WEXLER

_____

INSURANCE CARRIERS, LTD

_____

Appendix **D**

Cash Reserve Release and Terminal Liability Agreement

This Cash Reserve Release and Terminal Liability Agreement, effective February 1, 1986, is between Davison, Donohue, and Wexler (Policyholder) and Insurance Carriers, Ltd. (Carrier).

Policyholder has established a limited liability plan under which the majority of health and dental coverage is self-insured; the remainder is insured under Group Policies GPZ-1022 and GPD-Z1022 (Policies). In consideration of Carrier's return to Policyholder of the Policies' extended liability cash reserves for health and dental coverage, Policyholder agrees to obtain an irrevocable bank letter of credit in Carrier's favor to serve as a reserve for extended liability in the event of termination of the Policies. Policyholder and Carrier further agree as follows:

1. Policyholder shall select a bank to issue an irrevocable bank letter of credit in Carrier's favor in the amount of Carrier's extended liability reserve requirements under the Policies.

    1.1   Carrier shall have the right to approve such bank and any letter of credit.

    1.2   Any charges made by the bank in connection with the letter of credit shall be paid by Policyholder.

2. When an acceptable bank letter of credit has been received, Carrier shall prepare the statement of experience prior to April 1, 1986, for the Policy period January 1, 1985, to February 1, 1986, and return the Policies' unused health and dental liability cash reserves to the Policyholder.

3. Where no satisfactory replacement or extension of the bank letter of credit can be made prior to the expiration of such letter of credit, Policyholder shall transfer cash to Carrier in the amount of Carrier's requirements under the Policies not to exceed the letter of credit amount within 10 days of notice, or Carrier may draw any amount up to the face value of the letter and hold such security of claim reserves.

4. Carrier will prepare an annual Policy Statement of Experience which will show:
    4.1 Any increase in extended liability health and dental reserve requirements
    4.2 Whether any surplus from the preceding Policy period:
        4.2.1 Was used to offset prior Policy deficits
        4.2.2 Will be returned to Policyholder to be used to increase the bank letter of credit to satisfy Carrier's additional health and/or dental requirements
        4.2.3 Will be returned to Policyholder as a cash refund

5. Future Policy renewals will be on an incurred-claims (not a paid-claims) basis.

6. Future Policy Statements of Experience will be on a paid-claims (not an incurred-claims) basis.

7. In the event of termination of the Policies, Policyholder shall transfer cash to Carrier in the amount of Carrier's health and dental reserve requirements within 10 days of notice, or Carrier may draw any amount up to the face value of the letter of credit for required extended liability reserves and accumulated deficits. The Policyholder's liability shall not exceed the amount of the bank letter of credit plus any excess premium for the policy year payable to Carrier or available for benefit payments in the Transfer Account.

8. The liability of Policyholder shall be governed by the terms and conditions of the Policies and this Agreement.

9. This Agreement shall automatically terminate and Carrier shall release claim to any unused portion of the Letter of Credit or return any unused reserve to Policyholder only at such time as

Policyholder's liability to Carrier under the terms and conditions of the Policies and this agreement shall terminate.

DAVISON, DONOHUE, AND WEXLER

_____

INSURANCE CARRIERS, LTD

_____

Outline of Coverage Effective January 1, 1989

Life Insurance

$5000 for all eligible employees.

Medical Insurance

	Preferred providers	Other providers
Calendar Year De-ductible	Individual, $100 Employee plus one dependent, $200 Family, $300	Individual $250 Employee plus one dependent, $500 Family, $750
	Carrier will pay 80% of the first $7500 per individual ($15,000 per family) of eligible charges.	Carrier will pay 70% of the first $7500 per individual ($15,000 per family) of eligible charges.

Lifetime maximum benefit of $1 million.

Percentage of Costs Paid by Insurance Company (After Deductible)

	PPO	Non-PPO
Covered physician charges	80%	70%
Covered inpatient hospital room and board, and covered hospital miscellaneous charges	80	70
Outpatient services	80	70
Second surgical opinion	80	70
Diagnostic X ray and lab	80	70
Speech pathology	80	70
Physical therapy limited to 60 days per disability and a calendar year maximum of $1000)	80	70

Preventive

	PPO	Non-PPO
Well-baby procedures and immunizations are covered up to the first 2 years of life	80%	Not covered

Mental Illness, Substance Abuse, and Alcoholism

	PPO	Non-PPO
Inpatient facility (up to 45 days per calendar year)	80%	70%
Physician visits (maximum reimbursement of $1000 per year)	50	50

Lifetime maximum benefit of $50,000

Prescription Drugs

$5 per *brand-name* or $3 per *generic* prescription when using a preferred pharmacy (A *prescription* is a 34-day supply or 100 pills, whichever is less.)	When using any other pharmacy, the $250 deductible and 70% coinsurance will apply.

Spinal Skeletal Treatment (Subject to Deductible)

Limited to $10 reimbursement per visit
1 visit on any one day
50 visits during any one plan year

Home Health Care and Hospice Care

100% if authorized by carrier in lieu of hospitalization

Dependent Coverage

Dependents include a spouse and unmarried children (including step-children or legally adopted children) from birth to age 19, or to age 23 if full-time students in an accredited school.

All eligible employees are covered for life, medical, and dental on a noncontributory basis.

Dependents must be covered for (1) medical and dental, (2) medical only, or (3) dental only.

Dental Benefits

I. *Preventive, basic, and major.*   The plan will pay 75 percent of reasonable and customary costs for all eligible preventive and basic procedures. Benefits will be paid at 50 percent for all eligible procedures. The maximum dental benefit is $1000 during a calendar year.

II. *Orthodontia.*   Benefits are subject to a $100 lifetime, per-person deductible. The plan then pays 50 percent of reasonable and customary costs for all eligible charges in excess of the deductible. The lifetime maximum orthodontia benefit is $750.

The final interpretation of any specific information discussed is governed by the policies and certificates of insurance. No rights accrue to any employee by any statement in or omission from this outline.

Cost-Containment Features

Precertification

All nonemergency hospital admissions and *all* surgical procedures not performed in a doctor's office must be precertified by the carrier. The *insured* is responsible for notifying the carrier's review office.

Failure to notify the carrier will result in a $500 penalty.

Emergency Hospital Admissions

For an emergency hospital admission, the insured individual, the doctor, a member of the family, or the hospital must call the carrier's review office within 24 hours after admission.

Maternity

A call to the carrier is required within 24 hours of admission.

Authorized Hospital Pays

The carrier review office will determine and authorize an estimated number of days of confinement. Days in excess of those authorized but not medically necessary will be refused for payment.

Second Surgical Opinion

A second surgical opinion may be required by the carrier's review office. When requested by the carrier's review office, the second opinion will be paid at 100 percent. If the second opinion is not obtained, the benefit for the surgeon's charge will be paid at 50 percent.

Rate Structure

	Medical Benefits	
	Active employees	Retired employees
Employee only	$ 92.37	$ 92.37
Spouse only	146.01	146.01
Children only	71.51	71.51
Spouse and children	217.47	217.47

	Dental Benefits
	Active employees
Employee only	$16.24
Spouse only	16.24
Children only	14.13
Spouse and children	30.36

All eligible employees are covered for life, medical, and dental on a noncontributory basis. Dependents may be covered for (1) medical and dental, (2) medical only, or (3) dental only.

Flexible
Benefits Plans

We arc pleased to introduce a new benefit option that will allow you to use pretax dollars to pay your dependent medical and dental premiums, to pay for health care expenses which are not reimbursed by our medical or dental plan, or to be reimbursed for dependent care expenses.

Overview

The flexible benefits plans will give you the opportunity to lessen the impact of health care or dependent care expenditures by using pretax earnings to pay for the following items:

1. Medical or dental insurance premiums
2. Unreimbursed Health care expenses
3. Dependent care expenses

Using pretax gross earnings to pay for one or more of those items may actually increase your take-home pay. However, the actual tax savings or liability must be figured on an individual basis. We cannot assume responsibility for any tax liability incurred by employees. An example of this new tax treatment of benefit costs (assuming a $100 per month deduction for dependent medical or dental premium) and the effect on your take-home pay under this new plan is shown on page 174.

Assumptions	Dependent benefit premium paid out of net (after-tax) pay	Dependent benefit premium paid out of gross (pretax) pay
Annual unadjusted gross pay	$15,000	$15,000
Monthly unadjusted gross pay	1,250	1,250
Pretax benefit contribution	—	(100) ($100 deducted for dependent coverage)
Monthly adjusted gross pay	—	1,150
Taxes (assume 20% of gross pay)	(250)	(230)
Net pay	1,000	920
After-tax benefits contribution	(100)	(—)
Take-home pay	900	920
Annual tax savings	—	240

You will be required to decide which of the three (3) parts of the flexible benefits plan you would like to participate in, prior to each plan year. You can participate in one or more options, or decline to participate entirely. If you choose to have your insurance premiums paid pretax, the payroll department will handle the administrative details for you. If you elect to participate in the health care or dependent care reimbursement account options, you will have to decide how much of your earnings will be directed to your account each year. Further details of each option are summarized below.

Medical or Dental Insurance Premiums

While the employer pays for the full premium cost of medical and dental insurance for most employees, the cost to cover dependents is paid by the employee. This cost is presently deducted from your net pay after taxes have been assessed. You can elect to have these premiums paid on a pretax basis by participating in the flexible benefits plan. Since federal and state taxes will not be assessed against these funds, your take-home pay may increase. If you make an election prior to each calendar year indicating your desire to pay premiums on a pretax basis, you will be eligible for this favorable tax treatment.

Medical FSA

The medical flexible spending account (FSA) will allow you to have a portion of your gross salary directed to an account established in your name which can be used to reimburse you for certain qualified medical care expenses. Each year you can elect in advance to have a specified dollar amount directed to a medical FSA. The amount directed to the account will be funded out of each of your monthly paychecks.

As you or your dependents incur certain health care expenses, you will pay the cost of the expense and then get reimbursed from your account with pretax dollars.

The types of medical expenses that are reimbursable are listed below.

1. Deductible and coinsurance payments from the medical and dental plans
2. Routine physical examinations
3. Vision care
4. Orthodontia care
5. Other health care expenses as allowed under pertinent IRS regulations and guidelines

Dependent Care FSA

If you have dependent care expenses that are necessary in order to enable you to work for the employer, you can direct a portion of your gross pay to a special dependent care FSA in your name. You will then be able to draw on this account to be reimbursed for qualified dependent care expenses on a pretax basis.

You can be reimbursed by the plan for the following expenses which enable you to work for the employer:

1. Care rendered to dependent children by a licensed day-care center or other facility or individual for which you are obligated to pay
2. Care rendered to dependent children or a spouse who is incapable of caring for himself or herself because of a physical or mental handicap by a licensed facility or individual for which you are obligated to pay

Outlined below are some questions and answers which should help to clarify most aspects of the plans.

How Do I Enroll?   Prior to the effective date, you must complete an enrollment form and forward it to the human resources department. You must choose how much to contribute to your medical FSA, dependent care FSA, or both. Also, you will need to elect whether your insurance premiums will be paid on a pretax basis. You do not have to choose what type of medical expenses will be reimbursed from your account until you file a claim. However, health care expenses can only be reimbursed from funds available in your medical FSA, and dependent care expenses can only be reimbursed from funds available in your dependent care FSA.*

Can I Change My Election During a Plan Year?   You can change your election during a plan year *if* you have a change in family status such as marriage, divorce, legal separation, birth or adoption of a child, or death of a dependent. Further, if your spouse has a change in employment status which affects eligibility under this plan, changes can be effected.

Do I Have to Make a New Election for Each Plan Year?   You must make a new election for each plan year to fund your medical and/or dependent care FSAs.

Is There a Limit to the Amount by Which I Can Reduce My Gross Salary to Pay for These Items?   Yes, the maximum by which you can reduce your gross salary is $5000 for the medical account and $5000 for the dependent care account (or $2500 per spouse if married and filing separate returns). The minimum annual contribution is $120.

What Happens to the Unused Account Balance at Year End?   Any funds left in either account at year end because they have not been used to reimburse you for eligible expenses are forfeitable to the employer. You must submit all final requests for reimbursement for claims incurred during a plan year within 90 days of the close of the plan year.

Can I Still Claim a Medical Expense Deduction on My Income Tax?   No, any amounts that you pay into the flexible benefits plan related to medical expenses are considered employer-paid medical benefits and are not tax-deductible. Most employees are, in any case, not able to take advantage of the medical expense deduction because their medical expenses do not exceed 7.5 percent of income.

Can I Still Claim the Dependent Care Expense Tax Credit?   No, to the extent that you pay for eligible dependent care expenses from your dependent care FSA, you will not be able to take advantage of the federal income tax credit for dependent care expenses.

---

*Note to reader: On January 1, 1990, this provision changed. Henceforth, medical FSAs will be treated like life insurance. The effect of this change will require the employer to advance the total amount to be reserved for 1 year even if the funds are not yet in the account.

Appendix **G** through **K**

Appendixes G through K present several strategic models that may be used by employers and insurance committees as a guide to planning and choosing medical benefits coverage for employees.

An employer's objective in an insurance study is to develop strategies for managing future increases in costs. Phases 1 and 2 provide the necessary background and documentation of cost-management difficulties to enable an employer to make an informed choice of an alternate insurance vendor and a PPO. This choice sets in place the basic strategic model I, which is described in Appendix G. Appendixes H through K describe further developments that employers may want to explore.

The responsibility for rising medical costs should be shared by employer, employees, providers, and government. An employer's budgetary restraints may prevent maintenance of benefits guarantees. If future medical plan increases substantially exceed general fund increases, the choices will be clear. The employer will be forced to make program or staff reductions, or employees will have to bear these costs, or providers will have to find more efficient ways to deliver services, or government will have to intervene.

If the employer is forced to offer additional plan options that increase financial pressure on benefits costs, employees may ultimately suffer the consequences. Medical care has advanced dramatically in the past 10 years, but whether it will continue to advance depends upon the available financing mechanisms. Unlimited coverage and multiple choices with minimal cost increases are naive expectations.

Efficient providers and management systems that control costs should be rewarded with more patients. Some employee dissatisfaction is to be anticipated, but it is a better alternative than erosion of needed financial protection.

Strategic Model I: Basic PPO and Indemnity Plan

Description

This model allows employees to choose between a managed PPO and an indemnity plan offered by a single insurer. Employee contributions, provider management, plan administration and or design (i.e., out-of-pocket expenses) may be used to modify future increases.

Impact

Increases in employer contributions needed to maintain employee coverage will probably continue to exceed increases in general fund.

Employee costs for dependent coverage, employer contributions for employee coverage, and higher out-of-pocket expenses will erode take-home pay.

Additional plan design changes may also be needed to offset premium increases. resulting in higher costs for employees who use the plan.

Employees will continue to be dissatisfied, and will become more involved in plan design and contribution decisions.

Comments

Plan design, administration, and/or contribution changes are directly related to increases in provider charges and or utilization of services. The employer will probably face 15 to 20 percent or higher increase in medical plan costs for 1990 unless current utilization management and provider price controls are effective. Further rises in plan costs will be caused by medical care providers who raise fees or changes, unbundle services, and/or perform more expensive or unnecessary procedures than a condition warrants. Subsequent-year increases will be based on the same factors that prevail in 1990.

Strategic model I is an employer's best short-term alternative, considering the changes occurring in the medical care system, the uncertainty over future premium costs, and the interest in maintaining employee contributions. This strategy is designed to stabilize costs and test the effectiveness of tighter utilization management and price controls on preferred providers. The results should be evident in 12 to 18 months. Additional plan options should not be added unless their impact is certain and unlikely to raise costs. The major determinants of future premium costs will be:

- Inflation (trend)
- Utilization
- Adverse selection

Inflation has long been blamed as the major cause of medical premium increases. But inflation means more than just increases in provider prices. *Medical care inflation* also encompasses increased use of technology such as new equipment or procedures and increased access to medical care.

An employer can reduce unnecessary medical services through plan design (e.g., employee cost sharing), administration (preadmission review), and use of managed delivery systems (PPOs and HMOs). However, it would be very difficult and perhaps inappropriate for an employer to try to directly influence use of, or access to, new medical technology by employees. This remains the realm of providers and utilization managers. And the prices of medical care service—i.e., physician charges and hospital billed charges—remain in the province of the providers.

The medical care market is being divided into different pricing arrangements. The traditional fee-for-service medical system is shrinking PPOs and HMOs are capturing an increasingly greater share of the employer and employee market. Substantial pressure is being brought to bear on normal physician fees and hospital charges, as HMOs and PPOs demand and receive discounts previously not seen in the fee-for-service system. This has resulted in at least a two-tiered system of fees and charges.

The traditional fee-for-service system is a full-priced retail system with uncontrolled rates of increase. The HMO/PPO managed care system is a discounted price system with annually negotiated increases. Whether the discounts will actually result in long-term savings is uncertain, because providers may develop methods to counter these discounts. If prices are principally controlled by providers, employers' efforts should concentrate on controlling utilization and selection.

New types of carriers' agreements that include managed care and PPO arrangements have greater potential for success than traditional indemnity plans. Pushing through additional changes prior to stabilization of the current plan costs would make future strategic decisions more difficult. In the meantime, increasing employee cost sharing to reduce utilization and to exert downward pressure on providers' ambulatory services fees is the best strategy for the employer.

Cost sharing is an effective way to increase employee awareness of and sensitivity to consumption of minor medical services. The employee survey indicated that employees placed highest value on catastrophic protection. Cost sharing provides the best assurance of preserving catastrophic protection by reducing usage and the costs allocated for management of medical services. The question remains whether continued increases in costs will create a level of cost sharing that threatens the financial protection employees need.

The current out-of-pocket expense level won't bankrupt most employees. The question with a cost-sharing strategy is whether total costs can be sufficiently controlled to prevent the shifting of major financial burdens onto employees. If health care costs are not controlled and do not soon begin to conform closely to general inflation rates, the single remaining solution will be government intervention in the form of price controls and rationing.

Strategic Model IA: Basic PPO and Indemnity Plan with HMO Option

Description

Strategic model IA offers an HMO as a third alternative to the strategic model I choice between a PPO and an indemnity plan.

Impact

Employees receive a comprehensive care alternative to traditional fee-for-service and PPO delivery options.

A prepaid concept of financing care is introduced as an alternative to the PPO or indemnity cost-shared approach.

Employees will probably be required to contribute for HMO coverage.

Potential for adverse selection and increased costs for the employer's indemnity and PPO plans is created, especially if the HMO plan experience and premium rates are not combined with other plans offered by the employer.

Comments

Employers may face 15 to 20 percent or higher increases in PPO and indemnity plan costs, on average, for 1990. Further PPO and indemnity plan design changes that increase employee cost sharing may increase pressure for an HMO alternative.

The company may be expected to fund the higher cost of the HMO option. The HMO will be the highest-priced option ($120 to $150 for the premium for each employee) because it will have the most comprehensive benefits.

Addition of an HMO may have adverse impact and may require higher prices for the PPO and indemnity options. The organization may be asked through negotiations to fund these higher costs. Using one carrier for all three options can help control the premium prices for the plans.

This strategy continues the current PPO and indemnity plan options and offers an HMO as a third alternative. This gives employees a comprehensive first-dollar care alternative. The prepaid approach gives employees a method of financing comprehensive care in advance. The questions are: Will employees be willing to pay for these better benefits? What will be the impact on the other plans offered by the employer?

The HMO's comprehensive benefits are usually more expensive than indemnity and PPO plans, with significant cost sharing. Employees are required to pay the difference between employer contributions toward the indemnity or PPO plan and the HMO premium. The use of pretax payroll deductions continues.

Another issue that arises when an employer adds an HMO is its impact on both the employer's and the employee's costs for the indemnity and PPO plans. Theoretically, an HMO, with its internal controls, should be better able to manage care for less than the unmanaged fee-for-service system. It also should be more efficient than a less tightly managed PPO arrangement.

Studies show that some HMOs do achieve efficiencies in delivering care. However, premium differentials between HMO and non-HMO plans often do not directly reflect these efficiencies. Many times this is due to risk selection differences between the two plans. This can be a significant problem if the employer uses more than one insurance carrier and the relative value of the HMO plan is not reflected in premium costs.

HMOs that do not use an experience rating set premium costs based on community averages and the potential for selection occurs. Selection is the process by which employees choose the option most financially advantageous to their own situation. If adverse selection occurs, total employer costs will increase more rapidly than they would in the absence of a third alternative.

This situation can be best explained by an example. Say an employer has a combined indemnity and PPO plan with all employees insured at an average premium rate. All claims, whether indemnity or PPO, are pooled and paid from the premiums received. There are no premium differentials based on plan use or use of PPO or non-PPO providers. As costs have increased, employees have become more aware of premiums and how much they individually use the plan. Some—mostly low-use or no-use employees or individuals who have other coverage available— are looking for lower-cost alternatives.

During 1988 the employer's benefit program had employees with no claims, employees with low claims, and employees with large claims. The following table shows 1988 medical plan costs broken into three cost categories of employee and family usage.

Example: Medical Plan Cost Breakdown

Employee and family yearly usage	Amount paid in medical claims per year	Number of employees	Average monthly claims cost per employee
Over $5,000 in claims	$1,966,531	110	$1,490
Under $5,000 in claims	$1,743,904	2,028	72
$0 in claims	0	157	0
Total	$3,710,435	2,295	$ 135

Most employees and families with large claims (over $5000) cannot afford to pay the average monthly cost ($1490) of typical claims in their category. They rely on a fundamental principle of insurance called *risk sharing*. As in most group plans, employees with large claims are subsidized by employees with low claims or no claims. Herein lies the potential for selection against the employer's plan and the threat to future increases.

In 1988 the average medical plan cost per employee (including dependents) was $135 per month. The average monthly cost for high users was $1490, for low users it was $72, and for nonusers it was $0. If a community-rated HMO is allowed to enroll employees at a premium rate of $120 and the average cost of services per employee and family is only $72, the employer's enrollees will be subsidizing other nonemployer subscribers. If the HMO plan experience is not combined with the employer's indemnity and PPO plan financial experience, the employer will lose the positive effect of the low user group on its average cost. Average costs for those who remain in the indemnity and PPO plan will increase more rapidly.

Community-rated HMOs do not account for their premiums on the basis of actual costs of medical services used by each employer group. It is possible for an HMO to enroll 100 employees, collect $100,000 in annual premium, and deliver only $50,000 in services. The financial incentive for a non-experience-rated HMO is to attract low-use or no-use subscribers. The employer's incentive is to encourage its worst health risks to join the HMO. In the long run, either the employer or the HMO will lose and the financial relationship will become unsatisfactory.

The problems described above may be avoided by contracting for an experience-rated HMO that is combined with an indemnity and PPO plan, or perhaps by contracting for a separate stand-alone experience-rated HMO in which the employer controls employee contributions.

An HMO arrangement, to be worth considering, must be experience-rated. Full accountability is also essential. Most HMOs, except federally qualified ones, can meet these requirements. If the employer is mandated by a federally qualified HMO, which is currently prohibited from offering experience rating, accountability and experience rating will have to be negotiated.[*] The employer needs to remember that if plan prices reflect both the benefit differences and the risk-sharing protection provided by each plan, selection will adversely affect future costs.

[*]Federally qualified HMOs will be able to negotiate this within 2 years.

Strategic Model IB: Plan I or IA with Catastrophic Plan Option

Description

Strategic model IB upgrades either model I or model IA by adding a catastrophic plan option with a higher deductible ($750 to $1000), a higher out-of-pocket limit ($5000), and a lower copay (60 to 70 percent). Differences in cost between the catastrophic and the option I plans are to be paid to employees in increased pay or put into an FSA.

Impact

Employees who need less coverage or who are willing to take more risk are allowed a wider range of choices.

Employees who select only the catastrophic plan receive higher take-home pay.

Costs for the options in strategic model I increase more rapidly as low users opt for catastrophic coverage only. There is greater potential for adverse selection to affect the options in strategic models I and IA as younger, healthier, and otherwise covered staff choose catastrophic care only.

Comments

The employer's contribution may eventually cover only the cost of catastrophic coverage. This model adds another option, with higher out-of-pocket expenses to the indemnity or PPO plan. Its principal impact will be different premiums for high and low plan enrollees. Employees who need less coverage (e.g., those whose spouses also have coverage, or who are financially well off) or may be more willing to take risks (e.g., who are younger, who live a healthier, better lifestyle) will receive lower premiums. The result is that employees who stay with strategic model I (or the HMO if applicable) will pay higher premiums. Also, some enrollees may face substantial out-of-pocket expenses if accidents or other unpredictable medical expenses arise.

One advantage of this model is greater employee choice and equity based on plan use. Another is that a catastrophic plan introduces a higher level of employee cost sharing and awareness. A third is that it provides an alternative for employees who are primarily concerned about rising premiums.

The FSA still allows employees to fund expected unreimbursed medical expenses on a pretax basis. This may be more economical for some than joining the lower-deductible plan and paying a higher premium. The recently issued technical corrections to Section 89 require employers to reimburse employee expenses before they may be funded by the employee's FSA. This places an additional financial risk on the employer and may force discontinuation of the FSA option, thus taking away an incentive for joining the higher-deductible plan.

The financial impact of strategic model IB will be higher costs for strategic model I enrollees and lower costs for catastrophic plan enrollees. Total costs may increase slightly due to adverse selection, but this can be minimized if all plans are carried by one insurance company.

Lower-paid employees may be persuaded by lower premiums to enroll in the catastrophic plan, which could lead to economic exposure they may not be able to absorb. This could result in increased hardship cases among the employer's staff.

Strategic Model II: Employer-Paid Catastrophic Plan with Employee Purchase of Plan I, IA, or IB

Description

Strategic model II is useful when a large rate increase forces an employer to provide a fixed contribution that may only be capable of funding catastrophic coverage. The indemnity and PPO coverage is split into separate plans with separate costs. An employee can purchase a PPO, an indemnity, or an HMO plan, or can fund an FSA through pretax payroll deductions. The same carrier should be used for all plans.

In this model, there is a clearly defined employer contribution each year.

Impact

Employees may expect the employer contribution to be sufficient to maintain indemnity or PPO benefits, whereas the contribution may cover only the catastrophic plan or a high-deductible PPO.

The defined-contribution arrangement promotes a total compensation concept.

Staff are given an opportunity to understand the direct relationship between coverage and costs.

Comments

Individual prices for each plan (i.e., catastrophic, PPO, indemnity, HMO) eliminate the egalitarianism of the single price structure. The impact of adverse selection increases but can be reduced somewhat by different prices for each plan and use of one carrier. The employer can better control its financial future by moving to a defined contribution and assuring that at least one or two plans fall within the limits of its contribution. From 1991 on, negotiations should focus on the amount contributed by the employer.

This model is substantially the same as strategic model IB, with the exception that the catastrophic plan becomes the base plan and employees choose additional coverage funded principally by their own contributions. Strategic model II may be the only practical solution for an employer if a large rate increase occurs, requiring substantial changes in the indemnity and PPO plan. With this plan, employer contributions will be more clearly defined and their rate of increase more clearly related to salary increases. Employees become totally responsible for their level of benefits protection and their contribution amount.

This model represents a substantial change in philosophy over the typical employer's past position. The insurance committee is expressing an interest in more options for employees if cost controls are effective and premiums don't continue to increase faster than wages. The employer gets better control over its costs and more visibility for its contributions. The employer can further promote the total-compensation concept by defining its contribution in dollars toward benefits. This cafeteria-style plan provides the freedom of choice many employees favor. The major drawback is that employees must fund their protection needs directly from salary. This is a harsh reality many may not be prepared to accept. If an employer chooses this model, its incremental step toward full flexible benefits is rather small.

Strategic Model III: Full Flexible Benefits

Description

Strategic model III differs considerably from defined-benefits plans in that it is a defined contributions plan. It offers multiple plan options, including cash. Employees are free to purchase from a variety of medical plans. Among the options are an HMO, catastrophic coverage, high-indemnity, low-indemnity or PPO plans, either a high-coverage or a low-coverage dental plan, a vision plan, and an FSA. Trading vacation pay and/or sick leave for coverage may also be a possibility.

The employer is required to make contributions to fund benefits at a higher level and at a higher percentage of pay than in the past.

Impact

The implied employer "maintenance-of-benefits" guarantee is replaced by an employer defined-contribution policy with higher funding.

More money is available for FSA or increased take-home pay as options.

Increased plan administration and increased communication with employees are required.

Employees' pressure on the employer to maintain benefits is transformed into pressure for more pay or flexible benefit dollars.

Comments

The employer's involvement with the carrier and the broker-consultant will increase because of the need to deal with more complex plan pricing and plan designs. Employees' selections and reduced risk pooling will move the cost burden toward higher-utilization employees who have higher risks. Adverse selection and administration will raise the total plan costs.

Individual plan prices will more directly reflect benefits plan usage, as well as employees' willingness to trade salary and other benefits (e.g., vacation) for health care benefits. Differential prices should cause employees to weigh annual enrollment decisions more carefully. Dissatisfaction usually results among the high users of medical plans and among the employees who need the highest levels of financial protection.

Strategic model III, incorporating full flexible benefits, requires increased employer funds for benefits. The employer will need to define its contributions policy and to offer multiple plan options, including the option to trade benefits for increased pay or more vacation. The options offered will include an HMO, catastrophic coverage, high- and low-indemnity and PPO plans, a high-coverage and a low-coverage dental plan, a vision plan, and an FSA. Trading of vacation pay and/or sick leave may also be included to provide more dollars for funding medical plan treatments.

This model is a dramatic change from more traditional plans, and requires a substantial increase in either the employer's or the employee's ability to fund benefits. More funding permits employees to have more choices and increased ability to satisfy divergent individual needs. This should result in increased employee satisfaction. Higher costs will be paid by high users, a situation which may in time erode these employees' satisfaction or understanding if their ability to finance plan choices does not keep pace with costs.

Flexible benefits cause employees to focus their efforts to pressure the employer on pay. Flexible benefits provide the employer with a way to fix or index cost increases. The increased complexity and freedoms allowed by flexible benefits require more administration and communication from the employer. Greater reliance on the carrier, outside consultants, and/or broker-consultants will be needed.

Whether or not adoption of full flexible benefits will represent a realistic option for the employer or will be fully understood by employees is uncertain. Flexible benefits provide the employer with a solution for cost increases while also providing improved benefits to employees. The employers' limit on its contribution costs may be interpreted as shifting the burden of future medical care increases onto employees. Whether or not the incremental value of offering employees more choices will justify increased costs for employees, more complex plan administration, and potential misunderstanding depends primarily upon whether the employer and the employees have the funds to finance such a benefits change.

Glossary

Administrative Charges: Costs, included in a carrier's retention fee for a medical benefits package, which cover such administrative services as bookkeeping, overhead, company newsletters, and conferencing with insureds.

Administrative Services Only (ASO): A contract with an independent insurance consultant or administrator for services that may include claims processing, case management, and accounting functions. This type of contract is sometimes chosen by employers that have self-insured programs. (*See also* Broker-Consultant; Independent Consultant; Third-Party Administrator.)

Adverse Selection: Choice of a program that allows high utilization of provider services by employees with high medical needs, when employees may choose from among several plans. Healthier (often younger) employees tend to select an HMO or other program that meets their needs as low users of medical services. As a result, the costs associated with the plan selected by employees with frequent utilization will outpace contributions, since too few healthy employees are enrolled to offset the frequent users of the plan.

Benefits Management Specialist: A staff member hired for the purpose of providing a medical benefits program to employees. The benefits specialist serves as liaison between employees and the insurance carrier, and is also involved in case management and education.

Bidding: The process by which a company seeks a health care insurance company. During the bidding process, carriers submit detailed explanations of the cost of the program, the premiums, and the services they can provide based on the bid specifications of the company.

Broker-Consultant: A person who acts as liaison between a company and its health care provider. Broker-consultants typically work for national firms that provide consulting and actuarial services as well. Many consulting firms maintain offices throughout the United States and bring a national perspective to their interpretation of a company's insurance situation. (*See also* Administative Services Only; Independent Consultant; Third-Party Administrator.)

Capitated Fee: A flat fee accepted by a physical for each person enrolled in his or her plan.

Carrier: An insurance company that provides group policies.

Carve-out: A claim made by an insured to a second carrier after receiving benefits from the primary carrier. The second carrier can refuse to pay any benefits if the insured has already received higher benefits from the primary carrier than the second carrier would have paid if it had been the primary carrier. (*See also* Coordination of Benefits.)

Case Management: The practice of planning, reviewing, authorizing, and evaluating an individual insured's case with regard to a specific illness or procedure or a series of illnesses and procedures.

Catastrophic Coverage: The total amount of coverage available to an employee for a particular illness. It is usually considered to be the maximum lifetime benefit amount. Insureds having only catastrophic coverage usually have deductibles of $5000 or more.

Claims Experience: The number of incurred and paid costs of claims filed by an individual or group in a given plan year.

Claims Office: A central location where employees submit claims to be paid.

Copayment: Payment by an insured of a flat fee for any visit to a physician or provider. Such fees are often between $5 and $20 per visit. Copays are most frequently found in HMO, PPO, and EPO arrangements.

Code Creep: The practice of escalating the coding of examinations that were previously coded as "brief" up to "limited," or "limited" up to "intermediate," and so on through "extended" or "comprehensive." This results in higher billed costs per unit.

Common Procedures Terminology (CPT): The names and codes given to specific procedures. Providers' bills are billed by code.

Community-Rated Plan: A plan in which premiums are based on the claims experience of everyone insured by the plan, including employees of several companies. (*See also* Experience-Rated Plan.)

Concurrent Review: Ongoing review of an individual's medical treatment by an agency or person other than the provider.

Coordination of Benefits (COB): Payment of the majority of a claim by a primary policy and the remaining by a second carrier. Typically the primary policy is offered by the person's employer, the secondary policy by the spouse's employer. (*See also* Carve-Out.)

Cost Shifting: The practice of requiring employees to pay a portion of the cost of medical insurance.

Deductible: A yearly amount that must be paid by an insured for medical care before the insurance carrier will begin paying a portion of the insured's total medical costs. (*See also* First-Dollar Coverage.)

Exclusive Provider Organization (EPO): A number of independent physicians, or a medical group, who enter into an arrangement with an insurance provider whereby they supply all medical services needed by the provider's insureds. Insureds enrolled in an EPO may use only those doctors and must designate one physician as their primary doctor. All other physicians must be seen by referral.

Experience-Rated Plan: A plan in which the cost of the premium is determined by the costs of the total group. Medical care, as paid out by the carrier, is totaled and added to the retention, reserve, and trend costs. The gross amount is then divided by the total number of insureds to arrive at a premium. (*See also* Community-Related Plan.)

Extension of Benefits (EOB): Continued coverage for individuals who are disabled at the time of termination of a plan. The length of time during which EOB applies is determined by contract language. This coverage applies only to disabled insureds who have no other coverage. The definition of *disability* can vary from one plan to another but typically means inability to work.

First-Dollar Coverage: Payment of medical claims without a deductible. (*See also* Deductible.)

Flexible Spending Accounts (FSA): An account into which an employee may deposit funds for later use in paying for a variety of medical and medically related services. At present, participating employees may deposit pretax dollars into their FSAs and later use them for medical services.

Fully Funded Program: A program in which an employer pays a predetermined premium to the carrier, who is then responsible for all costs incurred under the plan. If costs exceed the paid premium, the succeeding year's premium is increased to cover the loss.

Incurred but Not Reported (IBNR) Claims: IBNR refers to claims that are incurred prior to the end of a policy period but have not yet been filed.

Independent Consultant: A person who acts as liaison between a company and its health care provider. An independent consultant is usually affiliated with a local firm that does not maintain offices throughout the country. An independent consultant can perform many of the same services provided by large consulting firms but usually does not have the national perspective of a large consulting firm. (*See also* Administrative Services Only; Broker-Consultant; Third-Party Administrator.)

Independent Physicians Association (IPA): An association of physicians with varied specialties who practice within the same geographic area. IPAs represent their members in lobbying and contracting efforts. (*See also* Preferred Provider Organization.)

Loss Ratio: The difference between plan usage and paid premiums, expressed as a ratio.

Mandated Health Coverage: Certain insurance benefits that must be extended to all insureds, according to state or federal requirements.

Master Contract: A document that spells out all funding arrangements, eligibility requirements, coverages, and claims procedures for a particular insurance plan.

Maximum Medical Lifetime: The ceiling amount of available insurance for a particular insured individual.

Maximum Termination Liability (MTL): The maximum liability of the policyholder. Under this provision, the carrier cannot ask the policyholder for additional funds following contract termination, even if the IBNR and EOB claims exceed the reserves.

Minimum Premium Contract: A partially self-insured plan. The employer can contract with a carrier to provide a specific coverage. The employer pays a minimum premium to the carrier and maintains three benefits accounts: one for retention, one for medical claims, and a third for reserves. The employer can be responsible for costs exceeding the premium, depending on the type of termination liability.

Preferred Provider Organization (PPO): A group of physicians who have contracted with an insurance carrier to provide services to the carrier's clients at a specific fee. The insured is free to go to doctors outside the PPO network, but will not benefit from the price arrangement negotiated with the PPO. Insureds enrolled in a PPO can use any physician's service they choose as long as that physician is part of the PPO. (*See also* Independent Physicians Association.)

Providers: Physicians, medical technologists, physical therapists, and others eligible to provide services to patients under the master contract.

Reasonable and Customary: An evaluative phrase often used by insurance carriers in determining the amount they will pay on claims. The decision is based on what is considered to be the reasonable and customary fee in that geographical area for the service provided.

Reserve Account: A fund used to pay IBNR claims after the plan year ends and to pay claims by individuals who are covered under EOB provisions after the plan is termined. (*See also* Extension of Benefits; Incurred But Not Reported.)

Stop Loss: The point at which an insured's benefits will begin paying 100 percent of covered charges up to the maximum benefit.

Third-Party Administrator (TPA): A person or organization retained by a self-insured or partially self-insured program to oversee and coordinate claims administration for the benefit plan. (*See also* Administrative Services Only; Broker-Consultant; Independent Consultant.)

Trend: Medical care inflation. Trend comprises several factors: the rise in the medical consumer price index, cost shifting and averaging of costs, new advances in medical technology, and increased utilization of medical care services.

Unbundling: The practice of itemizing and billing for procedures and supplies that were previously billed as one item.

Index

About the Authors

MARY F. CALLAN has been a high-level player in the human resources arena for more than thirteen years. She is a pioneering activist in designing cost-effective health benefits packages and gaining their acceptance by employers, employees, their unions, local government officials, and the insurance companies. Dr. Callan is currently assistant superintendent of human resources, business, and strategic planning of the Beaverton Public School System, Portland, Oregon, and former executive director of human resources of a large Colorado school district.

DAVID C. YEAGER, a graduate of the University of Colorado, is a communications specialist who has written extensively on the subject of health care. He has received special recognition for his work in creating business-education partnerships in Colorado.